BACH FLOWER

REMEDIES FOR MEN

STEFAN BALL

BACH FLOWER REMEDIES FOR MEN

INDEX COMPILED BY LYN GREENWOOD

Saffron Walden
The C.W. Daniel Company Limited

First published in Great Britain in 1996
by The C. W. Daniel Company Limited
1 Church Path, Saffron Walden,
Essex, CB10 1JP, England

ISBN 0 85207 302 X

Design and production in association with
Book Production Consultants plc, 25–27 High Street,
Chesterton, Cambridge, CB4 1ND
Printed and bound by WSOY, Finland

For James Ball
and Fred Woodham

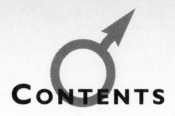

CONTENTS

ACKNOWLEDGEMENT

The vast majority of books list a single author on the spine and he or she takes all the credit. But even the most solitary of authors is trying out ideas on a host of other people and getting ideas, information and raw material in return. I'd like to thank everyone who helped me in this way, especially the ones whose names I can't remember or never knew.

Most of all I want to thank my wife Christine who read the whole manuscript from cover to cover and saved me from several errors and at least one serious embarrassment. Any of either that remain are of course my fault alone.

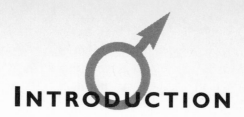

INTRODUCTION

SOCIAL PRESSURES

Imagine this: your seven-year-old daughter sees a ballet on television and says she wants to have lessons. What do you do?

Now imagine this: your seven-year-old son has seen the same television programme and he wants dancing lessons as well. What do you do now?

It's a measure of how far we have come and how confused we remain that the answers which would once have seemed obvious – encourage the girl and discourage the boy – are no longer obvious, but obviously problematic. Why should boys and girls be treated differently? What do we mean when we say 'be a man'? What is a 'man' anyway?

There is in fact little agreement about what men are, or about what it is that makes them different from women. According to John Nicholson, author of the book *Men & Women*, the weight of recent evidence tends to show that both sexes think and act in very similar ways. It seems that the only real distinction to be made is in the shape and function of the genitals and the fact that men cannot bear or give suck to children. Yet in every society and every culture little boys are treated differently from little girls so as to reinforce a particular stereotype of what a boy – and what a girl – should be.

In the case of male children the stereotype demands that they be strong and do not show emotion: boys don't cry. It is assumed that they will like or at least tolerate fighting and violence; perhaps this is why on average mothers hit their boys three times more often than they hit their girls. They will be given to climbing trees and pushing and shoving and playing cowboys and Indians. They will not be too neat and tidy. They will be risk-takers, so that chancing paralysis on the rugby field is an acceptable childhood activity (much more so than ballet) as is, to a lesser extent, potential brain damage in the boxing ring. As boys grow into men they are expected to be stronger, more independent, and more interested in sex and violence than in love. They will be hard and ruthless. They will compete for the most attractive women, the biggest cars and the highest-status jobs. In their maturity they will continue to show little emotion but will apply rational analysis to problems and come up with solutions irrespective of personal feelings or consideration for others.

The results for women of such ways of thinking are well documented. They may include a lack of job opportunities, fewer and less well-defended civil rights, reduced self-esteem and poorer self-image. It is perhaps less apparent that men too are victims of the process.

Nicholson recounts an experiment in which a group of American boys and girls between the ages of 8 and 14 was shown film of a baby lying in a cot. The heart-rates of both boys and girls slowed when the baby smiled – and sped up when the baby cried. Yet while the girls showed open interest in the film the boys feigned indifference. It isn't difficult to imagine the emotional, spiritual and physical cost of keeping up this pretence over a whole lifetime. As these boys grow into men they will be less able to share their problems and worries with others; they will smoke and drink and resort to drugs more often than women; they will suffer more from heart disease and other stress-related illnesses; they will have higher blood pressure; they will consult their doctors less, of course, since concern for one's health is not a manly trait; and unsurprisingly they will end by dying, on average, six years before their wives do.

THE 38 BACH FLOWER REMEDIES

'How many folk can you number amongst your friends or relations who are free? How many are there who are not bound or influenced or controlled by some other human being? How many are there who could say, that day by day, month by month, and year by year, "I obey only the dictates of my Soul, unmoved by the influence of other people?"'

These lines come from an address given by Dr Edward Bach to an audience in Southport in 1931. Today as then, freedom – the freedom to be yourself and to allow freedom to others – can only be gained by understanding and accepting who you are. What is needed is self-knowledge, the attainment of a very personal balance within the personality – also the strength to resist the distortions of other people's ideas and the pressure to conform to external standards of success and failure. There is no place in this vision for sexual stereotyping: instead of learning to be a 'man', men need a chance to be themselves.

Dr Edward Bach was a bacteriologist at University College Hospital and a researcher of some repute. But he slowly became disillusioned with orthodox medicine until in 1930 he abandoned his Harley Street practice to begin the search for a new and more natural way of treating his patients. His great insight – which came at a time when conventional medicine was becoming more reliant on technology and surgical intervention – was that physical health depended upon the emotional health of the individual. Consequently he looked for a way to treat emotional imbalances rather than physical symptoms, reasoning that if the mind and spirit could be cured the body would find its own equilibrium.

The 38 Bach Flower Remedies that we know today are the result of that search. Each one is directed at an emotional, mental or spiritual state. Together they make up a comprehensive and complete system that is simple to understand and can be used safely by anyone. You will learn more about the 38 Remedies as you read through this book, but for ease of reference they are listed here in alphabetical order, along with the main indications for each one.

AGRIMONY

This is the remedy for people who hide their worries and mental torture behind a happy, smiling face. They tend to be gregarious, fond of company and parties, and reluctant to come to terms with the more unpleasant side of life. The Agrimony remedy helps such people, or anyone who falls temporarily into such a state of mind, to face their troubles. Then, by seeing things in true proportion, they can build a cheerful outlook on firmer ground.

ASPEN

Aspen is the remedy for fearful feelings that do not have any known cause. Forebodings, feelings of impending disaster or the vague feeling that something frightening is happening all come under this heading. Also included are specifically uncanny fears associated with particular places or events and superstitious fears of all kind. The Aspen state is different from the Mimulus state, when the fear is of something specific that can be named.

BEECH

Intolerance is the key characteristic for Beech type people. They tend to be hyper-critical of other people's lives and take little thought for the circumstances which may have led others to live the way they do. But all of us at one time or another fall into a Beech state. When you find yourself wondering why other people insist on being less wise, less witty, less charming and less efficient than you, you could probably benefit from a dose of Beech.

CENTAURY

The Centaury man is the one who always seems to be at the beck and call of others. He seems quite incapable of standing up for himself. If he is unlucky enough to fall under the domination of a stronger character, he can find himself turned into a virtual slave. This is a shame, for at heart he is a good friend and willing helper who only needs a little help to say 'no' now and again. The remedy can provide this support when it is needed, just as it can for anyone who falls temporarily into this state.

CERATO

Cerato is the remedy for doubt in one's own ability to judge and to take correct decisions. Someone in a Cerato state will ask all and sundry for advice before deciding which way to go, even when he knows in his heart what it is he really wants. Buffeted by other people's willingness to help, he will lean in the last direction he was blown and may end up taking bad advice and feeling very stupid when (as he knew would happen) things turn out badly and his plans are scuppered.

CHERRY PLUM

Cherry Plum is used to restore mental balance whenever it is in danger of being overthrown by irrationality. Most men at some time or another know what it is to feel mental and emotional control ebbing away. The Cherry Plum state can be as simple as an emotional outburst or mild hysteria, and as complex and potentially dangerous as thoughts of hurting others or even of suicide.

CHESTNUT BUD

This is the remedy for those who seem unable to learn from past mistakes, and seem doomed to repeat them. The man who finds himself planning to repeat this Saturday the disastrous evening out he endured the Saturday before might benefit from the actions of this remedy. So might anyone who finds himself trailing a succession of failed relationships with similar people or an unrewarding series of similar jobs.

CHICORY

In their positive aspect Chicory people are full of love and care for those who are close to them. But in their negative aspect their love turns possessive and domineering so that instead of nurturing their loved ones they seek to control them and monopolise their time. The parent who feels slighted when his grown up children do not visit every week is a classic example of this type, but anyone who tends to cling and demand love and attention as a right is in this state, and may be helped by this remedy.

CLEMATIS

Clematis people are dreamers of great dreams. They love to drift off into hazy plans for the future. Unfortunately they risk losing any chance of turning their dreams into reality because they are not focused enough on the present to seize passing opportunities. The remedy helps keep the Clematis person anchored in the present so that the risk of this happening is reduced.

Because of their lack of interest in the present and in their surroundings, Clematis people may be particularly prone to drowsiness and can appear inattentive and withdrawn.

CRAB APPLE

Where someone feels unclean, is ashamed of his appearance, of medical problems or of how he has behaved, then Crab Apple is indicated. It is the cleansing remedy, and is effective as much against physical as mental uncleanness.

Crab Apple types can be prone to compulsive behaviour such as repetitive hand-washing, or checking and re-checking the same thing over and over again. They tend to focus too much on trivial matters; the remedy can be a great help in raising their sights to the truly important things in life.

ELM

Elm types are capable people who are normally self-assured and confident of their abilities. Because of this they are often entrusted with positions of responsibility. On occasion, however, a sudden feeling of inadequacy may shake their faith in themselves. When this happens the Elm remedy is indicated to help overcome any temporary weakness and restore the normal balance of the person's mind.

GENTIAN

This remedy is used to overcome those relatively mild feelings of discouragement and despondency that come as the result of a particular setback. Children downcast at an exam failure and employees failing to win a promotion could both benefit. Gentian is also often used to help people following a course of treatment who find that an apparent lack of progress causes them to lose faith and adopt a negative outlook.

GORSE

The indications for the Gorse remedy are similar to those for Gentian. In the case of Gorse, however, negative thoughts have grown deeper roots until the afflicted person feels that there is no more that can be done for him. He believes there is no point trying to improve matters and his mental attitude is one of hopelessness and despair. The remedy is used to fortify the spirit so that he can take up the struggle once more.

HEATHER

An over-preoccupation with himself is the main characteristic of the Heather person. He is the man at parties who blocks his hapless victim into a corner and talks for hours about his health problems, the things that happened to him, the things that he said and the things that he should have said. Dr Bach referred to Heather types as 'buttonholers' because they metaphorically (and sometimes literally) seize people by the buttonhole to keep them listening.

The Heather person's great fear is that he will be left on his own. Unfortunately his behaviour often causes the very loneliness he fears, since other people may start to avoid him. The remedy is used to turn his thoughts away from himself and out towards others so that he can listen as well as talk. When he is able to offer as well as take comfort he will find that other people are more willing to listen to him.

HOLLY

Holly is used to counteract the extremely negative emotions of hate, aggression, envy and suspicion. People in this state have forgotten how to relate positively to others. The remedy is used to restore them to themselves so that they can give generously and love well.

HONEYSUCKLE

Honeysuckle is the remedy for people who do not pay sufficient attention to what is happening now because their minds and hearts are fixed on the past. The remedy helps the afflicted person learn the lessons of the past without being held back by memories and nostalgia.

HORNBEAM

Hornbeam is one of the remedies used against fatigue. The Hornbeam state is often characterised as the 'Monday morning feeling' – lethargy and tiredness caused by the thought of getting on with a task. The cause of this general weariness is spiritual and emotional rather than physical (cf. Olive).

IMPATIENS

Impatiens is the indicated remedy for people who are always in a hurry. Impatiens people are quick in thought and deed and lose all patience with those who do not react as quickly as they do. The remedy helps to encourage a calmer attitude and so reduce the likelihood of nervous tension and stress-related illnesses caused by too much rushing around.

LARCH

Larch would be given to people who lack confidence in themselves. Larch types go through life predicting the failure of their every effort, and use this prediction as a reason not to try in the first place. As they do not try they are obviously bound not to succeed, so that the prediction of failure is a self-fulfilling prophecy. The remedy helps to remove the fear of failure so that the attempt at success can be made.

MIMULUS

Mimulus is for a fear whose cause can be named. The fear of public speaking, of losing one's job and of an aggressive dog would all be treated with Mimulus (cf. Aspen).

MUSTARD

This is the remedy used against those sudden black depressions that can afflict people out of the blue. If there seems no reason for feeling gloomy, if life is full of good things without a cloud in the sky, yet still feelings of despair and depression darken your pleasure in life, then Mustard is the remedy to choose.

OAK

Like the tree which provides the Oak remedy, Oak people are stout-hearted and strong. They shoulder responsibilities without a murmur and never spare themselves when it comes to working hard and helping others. Unfortunately these admirable qualities can lead them to keep plodding on with their tasks long after exhaustion and illness should have seen them confined to bed. At those times when the man of Oak works himself near to collapse the remedy is there to restore strength and a sense of proportion. Essential efforts can still be made, but without destroying the individual's health.

OLIVE

This is the remedy for people left exhausted and weakened due to some physical cause such as overwork, lack of sleep or a long bout of illness. Everything seems too much effort to people in this state, so they find themselves unable to take pleasure in life any more. The remedy helps to restore strength and vitality.

Olive is often given in conjunction with another remedy or remedies as part of a holistic solution.

PINE

This is the remedy against guilt. Sometimes the guilt is justified, as is the case with someone who is racked by thoughts of some bad action in the past. Other times it is unjustified, as with those people who needlessly blame themselves for the misdeeds of others. In both cases Pine is the correct remedy.

If you have done something wrong Pine will not give you back your clear conscience at once. But what it does do is allow you to learn from past mistakes. Instead of poisoning the rest of your life with useless regret you can learn to live with yourself and move on to a better future.

RED CHESTNUT

Red Chestnut people show extreme anxiety for the welfare of others, especially their loved ones. This can be debilitating not only to the worrying Red Chestnuts but also to the people they worry about. Their over-care, fussiness and negative thoughts about life can undermine people's confidence until they too feel anxious and inhibited. When the remedy is given to the person displaying Red Chestnut symptoms, the benefits are usually felt by a wider circle of people.

ROCK ROSE

This is the remedy for terror. The Rock Rose state could be seen as a stronger form of Mimulus or Aspen states. Either kind of fear – specific or unspecific – is best treated by Rock Rose when there is panic and terror rather than simple fear.

ROCK WATER

Rock Water people tend to have definite opinions and allow their beliefs to dictate the way they live their lives. If they fail to live up to their own high standards they can be very hard on themselves, and their over-concern with their own spiritual health can lead them to fanatical extremes of self-denial and mental rigidity. The remedy in this case is used to encourage a kinder and more humane mental state. High ideals are not discouraged by the remedy, of course, but the person is brought to realise that living a righteous life and the enjoyment of simple pleasures are not necessarily mutually exclusive.

SCLERANTHUS

The Scleranthus person suffers from chronic indecisiveness. If there are two possible courses of action he will vacillate between them until both time and the opportunity itself are lost. Similarly, the lack of balance in such people can lead them to experience sudden mood swings, so that they appear to be at the top of the world one minute and in the depths of despair the next. The remedy restores balance so that decisions can be taken rationally and promptly enough to take advantage of the moment.

STAR OF BETHLEHEM

The action of this remedy is to counteract the effects of shock. It is one of the key ingredients of Rescue Remedy (see below).

Shock is usually caused by a sudden event, so Star of Bethlehem is most often used when someone has just received unexpected bad news, been involved in an accident or had a fright of some kind. However, the effects of shock can linger long after the event. This remedy is just as effective when used against delayed effects as it is when put to emergency use.

SWEET CHESTNUT

The Sweet Chestnut remedy is indicated for people who are going through the most extreme kind of anguish and despair. It is particularly associated with bereavement, but it is indicated at any time when the future seems utterly black and without hope.

VERVAIN

Vervain people are nature's enthusiasts. They are fervent campaigners for social justice, committed perfectionists and inclined to pour themselves body and soul into any task they undertake. Their extreme mental energy can lead them to drive themselves too hard, however, and their ever-alert minds make rest and relaxation difficult to achieve. At times when the stress of the Vervain lifestyle is too much to bear the remedy is used to bring calm to the mental storm.

VINE

In his positive aspect the Vine person is a strong, confident and understanding leader. At his most negative he is a tyrant, riding roughshod over the needs and wishes of others, using his power in an arbitrary way and seeking to dominate rather than lead. Here as always the remedy washes out the negative aspects and replaces them with the positive ones. The Vine individual is restored to his natural balance and can assume rightful authority without deflecting other people from their own true paths.

WALNUT

Walnut is often referred to as the transition remedy. It is used to overcome any influences that might be getting in the way of following a particular path or making a particular change. The influences in question may be someone else's opinions, ties to the past or simply a habit acquired over time. In all cases Walnut helps to put the potential hindrances into perspective so that a balanced and true picture of the whole situation can be formed and a course of action decided on free of unwanted influences.

Walnut is commonly prescribed for all the normal changes of life, from cutting your first teeth to retirement, since it helps you to free yourself from old patterns of thought and embrace new states without regret.

WATER VIOLET

The Water Violet person is an intelligent, capable type who is happiest when keeping his own company. Although he is often admired by those around him, he can be thought proud and unapproachable, which means that he finds it hard to make friends and so can end up feeling lonely. The remedy is used to help such people unbend a little towards their fellow men so that, while they still enjoy their own company, they are able to call on others when they need to.

WHITE CHESTNUT

When a worry or unwanted thought intrudes upon the mind at all hours, or when you find yourself rehearsing the same argument over and over in your head, White Chestnut is the remedy to help. It works to check uncontrolled thoughts so that the mental processes can once more be constructive rather than destructive. Once it is under control, thought may be able to solve the root cause of worry rather than allowing the worry itself to take over.

WILD OAT

In some ways the Wild Oat condition is similar to the Scleranthus one, in that both are to do with uncertainty and indecision. But people in the Wild Oat state do not usually have any difficulty taking small decisions, and their uncertainty is centred on finding a goal worth aiming at rather than choosing which of two alternative methods will allow the goal to be reached.

Despite the fact that they want to make some definite contribution to life Wild Oat people are lost, and their great talents and many gifts do not help them make up their minds what that contribution should be, or even what alternatives are open to them. People in this state often try several different careers without finding one they can really commit to. The remedy helps them to define their own characters more successfully so that they can pick a direction and follow it with all their hearts.

WILD ROSE

Resignation and apathy are the watchwords of the Wild Rose person. This is someone who has given in to circumstances and makes no effort to change himself or his condition. If ill, he will make no effort to get well; if poor, he will shrug his shoulders and carry on drifting.

In either case he lacks any real interest in or commitment to life. The remedy is used to wake him up to his surroundings and to his potential so that he can contribute to his own development and to the world around him. He may still be happy-go-lucky, but he will be able to take control of his life when he has to.

WILLOW

Like Wild Rose people, those in the Willow state do not always make the best companions. They are not apathetic, but resentful, full of self-pity and unkind thoughts about other people, especially those who are happier or more successful than them. Nothing can be done to please Willow people, and every service performed for them is taken without gratitude and with much complaint.

The Willow remedy helps such people to see things more clearly and take responsibility for their own destinies. Instead of begrudging the joys of other people they can come to take genuine pleasure in them. In this way joy enters their own lives as well.

RESCUE REMEDY

Rescue Remedy is probably the best known of the Bach Flower Remedies. In fact it is not really a remedy at all but a mixture of remedies, made up as follows:

- Cherry Plum for loss of control
- Clematis for faintness
- Impatiens for agitation
- Rock Rose for terror
- Star of Bethlehem for shock

It will be apparent from its ingredients that Rescue Remedy is specially mixed to deal with emergencies. Whatever your immediate reaction to an accident, bad news or a worrying situation, Rescue Remedy will probably contain at least one remedy that will help you to handle your emotions. And its great advantage is that it is contained in one bottle, and so can be carried about easily.

Rescue Remedy is used in all kinds of situations when there is no time or opportunity to select remedies from the full range. It is often associated with nervousness (before an exam, for example, or when about to give a speech), accidents (when it can help calm onlookers as well as the victim) and minor injuries of all kinds.

Rescue Remedy is also available as a cream, and in this form contains an extra remedy: Crab Apple. As the cleansing remedy, Crab Apple gives the cream a special power against cuts, grazes, rashes and other skin problems.

SELECTING AND USING THE REMEDIES

Dr Bach's aim was to have a healing system that would be as simple to use as possible. Whenever you go to select a remedy for yourself or your friends you should take a moment to remind yourself of this, because it is all too easy to be too subtle and end up losing yourself in ramifications and theories that in fact have nothing to do with the matter in hand. Nevertheless there are a few simple concepts to be grasped if you are going to make a success of choosing the correct remedies.

The first thing to understand is the difference between type remedies and helper remedies.

A type remedy is the remedy (or, occasionally, combination of remedies) that best matches the individual character of the person being treated. For example, someone who is impatient at delays and tends to rush around all the time is probably an Impatiens type, while the strong, able man who plods on through every adversity is in all likelihood an Oak person. Once you know what someone's type remedy is you know which remedy is likely to be of use when that person encounters a problem, since a person's negative characteristics are usually at the root of the symptoms he complains of. The positive characteristics associated with each personality type and remedy are the qualities that flood in to take the place of these negative traits. For example, the positive side of Impatiens is a feeling of great calmness and serenity, and the aim of treating an impatient person with Impatiens is to encourage this side of his nature.

Despite the fact that a person's type remedy will remain the same throughout his life, most people experience at some time all 38 of the feelings and thoughts for which the 38 Bach Flower Remedies are indicated. This is because not only do we have a basic character type, which remains more or less constant, but we are also creatures of mood who can pass through a dozen different emotional states in as many hours. The Bach system allows for this, and all of the 38 remedies can be interpreted as helper or mood remedies. The word 'helper' indicates that when used in this way they are often chosen in addition to the type remedy itself. But in other cases, such as short-lived moods and transitory states, they can be given by themselves and without going into the why's and wherefore's. So if you suffer a panic attack you can reach for the Rock Rose without worrying too much about whether your type remedy is Clematis or Water Violet. But if you find you suffer panic attacks on a fairly regular basis you will need to give rather more thought to the underlying reasons for this – and many of these will be brought to light when you define your type.

As this last example shows, it is important when faced with any kind of chronic or recurring state to get below the surface of the problem, and the obvious symptoms so as to uncover the real underlying mental or emotional causes. These can at times be so deep-rooted that the individual is barely aware of them, but they are there all the same and, once they are known, the remedies can be used to produce a longer-term solution.

If selecting the remedies is best done with a little thought and a true understanding of the remedies, taking them is the simplest thing in the world. There are two main methods. Which you choose depends entirely on how persistent the problem is, and on how economical you want to be with the remedies.

The prepared bottles of Bach Flower Remedies sold in the shops are known as stock bottles. They contain a single concentrated flower remedy preserved in alcohol, and if possible they should be diluted before being taken. The quickest and easiest way to do this is to add two drops to a glass of water. If you are taking more than one remedy at a time add two drops of each one to the glass. Then all you do is sip from the glass at intervals (every few minutes in acute cases; every few hours if you are treating a longer-term and less dramatic problem).

Obviously this method is most effective for sudden problems. For long-term treatment you may find it simpler to make up a treatment bottle for yourself. All you need is a 30 ml dropper bottle – the kind with a built-in pipette, which you can buy from most large chemists – and some still spring or mineral water. Add two drops of each selected remedy to the clean, empty bottle, then top up with the water. Take four drops from the treatment bottle four times a day, either dropping them onto your tongue (being careful not to let the dropper touch your tongue) or adding them to a glass of water. The treatment bottle should last about two weeks, but after this the water will deteriorate and any mixture left should be discarded. You can make it last a little longer by keeping it somewhere cool, or by adding a spoonful of brandy or cider vinegar to the mixture.

As Rescue Remedy is a mixture of five different remedies, with slightly less of each individual remedy in the bottle, the dosage is different. In all cases where two drops of a single remedy would be added to a glass or a treatment bottle, give four drops of the Rescue Remedy stock.

You can take the remedies in other ways should you need to. They can be added to any other drink if water is not available, and in real need drops of the stock concentrate can be given neat. (Please remember however that the stock concentrate is preserved in pure brandy. You should be sensitive to any religious, moral or medical considerations that might apply in particular cases.) Finally, an external application can be a benefit in some cases, for example gently stroking Clematis or Rescue Remedy onto the wrists or temples of someone who has fainted.

THE BACH APPROACH TO HEALING

Dr Bach's search for a new healing system was built on the belief that health was natural and ill-health the result of a failure to live according to your true personality. He believed that mental, spiritual and emotional turmoil have their inevitable end in physical illness, and that there is no point in treating the latter alone if the root causes remain untouched.

The flower remedies that he found are all natural and non-toxic, and so gentle that they can be taken in conjunction with any other course of treatment, whether orthodox Western medicine or other alternative or complementary therapies. It is very important to stress however that they do not replace other more physical courses of treatment. In many cases (and despite occasional complaints to the contrary) the technology-rich medicine of the West is the best possible recourse. Where there is physical illness, physical methods are an important part of the medical armoury and are not to be lightly put aside. For this reason no responsible Bach practitioner will ever encourage you to go against the advice of your qualified medical practitioner.

But there is more to human beings than the body, and it was Dr Bach's great insight to understand the important role played by personality and emotion in dictating the course of disease. The Bach Flower Remedies are there to help bring calm to the mental storms that modern life provokes. Their gentle and natural power puts us back in touch not only with our inmost depths, but with the noble simplicity of nature herself. They can help to strip aside the pressures of peer-group and society so that we can truly be ourselves and in this way find peace.

ABOUT THIS BOOK

A trawl through any bookshop will quickly yield dozens of volumes on medicine, dozens more on complementary medicine, and as many again of both kinds aimed specifically at women. Sadly, and for whatever reason, men are not so well served. Most men remain in a state of lamentable ignorance about their own bodies and the kind of health problems that are peculiarly theirs. And they tend to show just as much ignorance when it comes to the health choices available to them.

My hope is that this book will cast a little light onto both areas. It follows a broadly chronological approach, tracing the different challenges faced by men as they go through the different stages of life. It also deals briefly with a range of specific medical conditions that are confined solely or largely to men. In all cases suggestions are made for using the Bach Flower Remedies to help resolve problems and overcome difficulties. As he works through the book the general reader will gradually build up a good understanding of the principles of remedy selection so that he will be able to apply these skills to his own particular situation. The examples given and the details of symptoms and prognoses should also be a help to more experienced Bach practitioners, who will I hope gain as much as anyone from the effort of reading.

CHAPTER 1

GROWING UP
IN A MAN'S WORLD

THE FIRST AGE OF MAN

Women are traditionally known as the weaker sex, but at birth this would appear not to be the case. In fact male babies tend to be ill more often than their sisters and although they are larger than girls they are also weaker and less mature. Even with today's well-equipped maternity wards and the latest medical techniques they are more likely to die in the early months.

Some say that the increased frailty and susceptibility to disease of baby boys is rooted in their maleness: being male is not a 'natural' state. This is because all human embryos are in fact female in the first few weeks of development, and it is only when the hormone testosterone is produced that specifically male sex development starts. The weakness might start even earlier, at conception, when the father's small and relatively information-poor Y chromosome joins with the mother's X chromosome to determine the child's future sex. Female embryos, who get a double set of coding thanks to their having received X chromosomes from both parents, not only escape peculiarly male problems such as haemophilia but seem also to be more resistant to all forms of mental and physical disorder.

In any case it seems that new-born boys might be more of a trial to their parents than girls. As well as their increased susceptibility to illness there is some evidence that males babies sleep less and cry more than female ones. They also feed more erratically, demanding the breast at shorter intervals and for longer. Anything that can help the new baby to settle down at night must then be welcome since by helping the new baby to sleep parents are creating a more relaxed and stimulating environment for him. Surrounded by happier adults he will himself be more alert and able to learn when he is awake.

Those baby boys whose sleep problems stem from the fact that they are on the go all the time and never seem to wind down might be classic Vervain types. They are great explorers and enthusiasts, and when they become interested in something they seem to be able to stay awake for as long as they want. Although these Vervain characteristics might seem wholly positive there can be problems where the child's mental energy causes him to keep going long after his physical strength is exhausted. In these cases the remedy helps to bring his life back into a reasonable balance.

Other babies demand endless attention before they will go to sleep. Parents who find themselves having to rock their child to sleep every night, or end up walking him around for hours because he cries when he is put down, might be dealing with a Chicory child. In their positive aspect these are loving children with a huge amount of affection to give, but their negative side can lead them to demand attention and endless displays of affection at all hours of the day and night. The remedy is given in such cases to help the child feel more secure about his parents' feelings for him so that he is less in need of reassurance. Most children probably go through some form of Chicory state at some time or other in their lives.

More common still is the simple fear of being left alone. Mimulus would be the first remedy to consider in such cases, since this is the remedy for known fears such as fear of the dark or fear of losing the parent. If the fear turns panic-stricken, or you suspect that the baby has been suffering from a nightmare, Rock Rose could be given instead. Babies spend 50 per cent of their sleep time dreaming, so the odd bad dream is to be expected. Tantrums and any similar loss of emotional control could be treated with Cherry Plum.

Just as some children seem never to sleep, others seem to sleep all the time. In fact a new-born baby can spend 80 per cent of his time sleeping without there being any undue cause for alarm. Even at nine months he will still be sleeping around 14 hours a day. But all the same some children are definitely drowsier than others and this may cause concern to parents. Children of the Clematis type are probably the most renowned for sleepiness, as they can drift off at any time and in any circumstances. In practice, and in the case of young children, it is not all that easy to tell a genuine Clematis state from the child's normal ability to fall asleep at the drop of a hat, but where sleepiness regularly gets in the way of activities that the child usually enjoys then the remedy could be tried. But if a normally active child seems unduly drowsy you should seek medical attention at once. While usually there will be nothing wrong, drowsiness can be symptomatic of several medical disorders that might need urgent treatment.

After four months or so the new boy will start the process of weaning, when he slowly turns from a milk-only diet to solids (although solids are a deceptive name for the mashed vegetables, puréed fruit and liquidised cereals that children start off with, as any parent who has had to clean the kitchen after mealtimes will tell you). Sometimes the transition to real food is made smoothly and without fuss, but for some children (and their parents) it can be a frustrating and upsetting experience.

Where the transition itself seems to be causing the problem, so that the child seems to be held back by his old patterns of life and is finding it difficult to break away, then Walnut is the remedy to give. Chicory might be needed to help those babies who see breast-feeding as a sign that they are the centre of attraction and resent the attempt to make them forego this pleasure. It allows them to relax a little and encourages the secure feeling that they are loved even when the outward physical show is not always on offer. Other children again may simply find eating solids an objectionable thing to do. They may pull faces when offered food, jerk their heads away when you try to feed them and spit out the contents of their mouths the first chance they get. Such children may benefit from Crab Apple, the remedy for people who feel disgust at themselves or at some necessary biological function – in this case eating.

As with drowsiness, so any long-term or severe problems with eating could indicate that there is some physical problem below the surface that needs to be addressed. If you are worried about a child's eating it is always best to consult your doctor even if it is only to reassure yourself that all is well.

Even when weaning goes fairly smoothly there are bound to be setbacks and reverses along the way. At such times another remedy, Gentian, can benefit parents and child alike. It is the remedy used to overcome any tendency to feel discouraged when things go wrong: it encourages optimism and the faith needed to try again.

Gentian (and Walnut) can also be a great help with the other major behavioural change that all babies go through: potty-training. Here again boys tend to develop slower than girls. They start potty-training later and take longer to learn how to control their bladders and bowels.

Some children might be disgusted and upset by the whole business, and for these Crab Apple would be given to overcome these feelings. This is fairly rare, however, and more usually children are fascinated by everything to do with the toilet so that the only role for Crab Apple might come if there is an accident at night, for example, or while out in public. Any guilt felt after such an episode could be treated with Pine, and the shock of the event eased with Star of Bethlehem.

Sometimes very young children can get so wrapped up in what they are doing that they put off going to the toilet until it is too late – Vervain might be called for to temper their enthusiasm, Impatiens to get them to slow down enough to think about things beforehand, or Clematis where they have slid off into a daydream and forgotten themselves. If the accidents become rather too frequent so that the child seems not to be learning the lessons of his experience then Chestnut Bud is the remedy to select. This can help the child to move on to the next stage of his development rather than repeating the same pattern of behaviour.

Bed-wetting can be a problem even after potty-training has been achieved. At seven years of age, for example, 20 per cent of children are still wetting their beds from time to time. Sometimes there will be a physical reason for this, and a child of 4, 5 or 6 who has never or hardly ever been dry at night should be taken to a doctor just to be on the safe side. But most of the time the problem will be psychological, especially if a child who has been dry in the past suffers a relapse. Look for any major changes in his life that may have upset him, like a change of environment or routine, for example, when Honeysuckle or Walnut might be the first remedies to consider. With a problem at home, such as the illness of a parent, try Red Chestnut or Mimulus. If there is family conflict, Rescue Remedy might be a good choice for the child, or Agrimony if he seemed to be suffering his fears in the night while appearing outwardly cheerful during the day. The adults responsible for the disturbance might need Willow or Holly. All of these are suggestions only, of course, since the individual characteristics and emotional state of the child (and his parents) always determine the final choice of remedies.

Most, if not all, of the problems dealt with so far could apply to girls as much as to boys. This reflects the reality that for pre-school children there is usually little weight given to gender as such, so that boys and girls will play together happily and (if allowed to by the adults overseeing them) with the same toys. In an ideal world, sex-stereotyping and all other pressures to conform would be resisted ever after and the child's personality would continue to be the main criterion for all choices. But the pressures that pre-school boys have faced so far are usually fairly mild compared with what happens when they start school.

SCHOOL DAYS

Boys start a new life the day they start school. For the first time they will find themselves valued by adults not for what they are but for what they can do, and for this reason competitiveness and winning will become more important. At the same time the most important influence and the arbiter of behaviour will no longer be their parents, still less their teachers or other youth leaders, but rather the group, the gang, their peers and equals: other boys.

Given the big step that starting school represents it is no surprise that many children can suffer from nervous upsets of one form or another, both before they start and in the initial settling-down period. At this time the Bach Flower Remedies can be a great help, as the following examples suggest:

- Where a child seems to be a prey to constant worries, White

Chestnut is the remedy to give him control over his unwanted thoughts.

- The boy who seems happy enough during the day but goes through mental torture at night or when he is on his own would be given Agrimony since this is the remedy for those who hide their troubles from others.
- If a child says quite openly that he is scared of going to school then Mimulus, the remedy for known fear, is the right selection to make. This remedy would also be chosen for those children who are by nature timid, quiet and prone to anxiety.

Boys of the Mimulus type are also among the most bullied. Prone to stammering and liable to turn bright red if they are asked to stand up and read something in class, they represent an obvious target. Centaury children too can suffer in this way. They are by nature kind and eager to please, but as they find it very hard to say 'no' they are open to exploitation by others. The clever child who spends his spare time doing other boys' homework may well be a Centaury type; the 'fags' in the public school system are institutionalised versions of the same mind-set. The remedy in this case helps the put-upon child to stand up for himself – not in any violent way, of course, but by giving him confidence and inner belief so that he can trust his ability to resist the undue influence of others.

Bullying is a far more common problem than is generally supposed, and despite the occasional well-publicised case involving girls actual physical assault and intimidation is still a mainly male phenomenon. Most men can probably think of an occasion in their own schooldays when they were either the victims or the perpetrators of bullying. In fact joining in with the victimisation of another boy is often the easiest way to avoid becoming a victim oneself. In these circumstances guilt can arise, and Pine is the remedy to help a boy take account of and learn from this emotion without allowing it to get a hold of him. It is also one of the first remedies to consider for the victims of bullying, for although it might be thought that they have nothing to blame themselves for victims often feel guilty and at fault. They reason that if they were not too different or too clever or did not possess whatever quality it is that sets them apart from others, then the bullies would pick another target.

The problem of bullying is made worse by a code of behaviour that leads victims to try to cover up the problem. The shame of being bullied is nothing compared to the shame of turning to a teacher for protection – and the thought of angry parents turning up at school to demand justice for their child will often be the victim's worst nightmare. Children are also well aware of the fact that the protection of adults is never going to be full-time. They know that sooner or later they will be alone again with their persecutors. The child who has got a bully into trouble can expect even less mercy than usual.

There are unfortunately no easy answers to this problem. The main thing the bullied child requires is thoughtful and constructive help from the adult world. If you are a parent and you suspect bullying, then, you should first try to gain the boy's confidence by telling him that you will not do anything unless he agrees to it. This should allay his fears of a blundering intervention on your part making things worse. Only then can you try to persuade him to let you talk to the school authorities about the problem. It is also a good strategy for the bullied child to try not to react to provocation and avoid situations where trouble is more likely. Boys in particular might feel that they should be squaring up to the challenge physically, and that by not doing so they are not behaving in a manly fashion, but in the real world bullies are usually bigger than their victims and tend to go around in groups. Fathers should remember this and avoid spontaneous self-defence classes and homilies on the need to stand up for yourself: encouraging a child to see violence as an answer to such situations is probably not a good idea. If a boy feels self-disgust at his weakness and inability to stop the bullying Crab Apple might help, and Larch is the remedy to help restore self-confidence. But probably the overriding emotion in the victims of bullies is sheer terror. Rock Rose would be the first choice to counteract this.

Bullies are usually no happier or secure in themselves than the people they pick on. Their bullying may be a way of bolstering a fragile sense of masculinity built on brute power and dominance and they may need help resisting the widespread idea that being a man is the same as being hard, tough and unfeeling. Walnut is the remedy to help people break free from the unwanted influence of their environment or the beliefs of others, but other remedies might also be appropriate in particular cases, for example:

- If the bully feels inadequate at home or at school, and bullies others to achieve some kind of status, then Larch is worth trying.
- If attacking others is an outlet for frustration at being held back, Impatiens is the remedy for these agitated feelings and mental pressures.
- Envy, jealousy and hatred are all countered with Holly.
- Boys whose bullying seems uncontrolled and frenzied, with little rhyme or reason behind it, might be helped by Cherry Plum.
- Beech is the remedy for intolerance of other people and is best used where the bully focuses particularly on people who are different from himself, his family, class or ethnic group.
- Vine is used to counteract aggressive behaviour founded on the desire to be top dog and dominate others.

The above examples show how bullying might be masking another problem in the child's life. It is necessary to define what the underlying problem is before the Bach Flower Remedies (or any other measure) can be used effectively. The real cause might be anything from fear and depression to a trauma caused by family illness, and the remedies needed will vary as widely.

Organised sport, so often praised as a panacea against misdirected aggression in schoolboys, can be a cause of humiliation and fear like bullying. In her book *The Rites of Man* Rosalind Miles recounts some truly gruesome sporting tales. These include the Welsh rugby master who split his class up into 'Large-Physique Boys' and 'Small-Physique-No-Talent Boys' and told the former to pick one of the latter and 'take him out'. Another example is the young Ernest Hemingway's first boxing lesson which ended with a nose broken in three places and a permanent injury to the sight of one eye. Organised sports (more correctly, badly organised sports) are occasions when spectacle wearers, asthma sufferers and the overweight are shown up as social outcasts and not 'real' boys at all. In small boys this kind of exclusion from their fellows is keenly felt, for the urge to belong to a gang, even if it is as the weakest member, is very strong. This is why boys accept dangerous or disgusting initiation ceremonies and dares as the price of entry to them.

The other condition for joining the all-male club (as well as being good at games) is that you have to be bad at emotions. Real men don't cry, goes the refrain from fathers, teachers (like the Welsh rugby master) and the media. Only women and cissies weep. Of course boys do have feelings, whatever society says; but they repress them in order to belong. The ones who are particularly good at doing so go on to develop a form of emotional autism that leaves them inarticulate and brutish. Inside they may be frightened and vulnerable, but outside they appear callous and indifferent. And the more frightened they are, the more likely they are to vent their anger and humiliation on others who have the courage not to be like them.

The roots of his later emotional problems undoubtedly lie in a man's schooldays, and it is then that any help given can be most effective. This help is needed not only because of the violent men that emotional autism produces but because of the loneliness, anxiety, stress and mental and physical illness that the inability to express emotion can lead to in later life. As the Bach Flower Remedies are specifically concerned with mental and emotional states they are particularly well-suited to help in this area. For example:

- Boys who hide their real feelings behind a smiling face could be helped with Agrimony.
- Rock Water would be indicated for boys who demand a great deal of themselves, following strict exercise or work schedules and sacrificing their gentler side on the way.
- Where attachment to order and control leads to intolerance of other people, Beech would be needed.
- Vine would be given to those who are power-hungry and inclined to the ruthless domination of others. Their lack of

compassion is rooted in their own emotional imbalance, so the cure for both lies in the same remedy.

- For those boys who fear the loss of self-control that might come if they are too free with their feelings, Cherry Plum is the indicated remedy.
- Fear of the emotions themselves would be a case for Mimulus.
- Where the emotions displayed are distorted by the need to conform to gang ethics, for example when a normally sensitive boy displays anger because that is what he is expected to do, then Centaury could be needed to strengthen his will to say 'no' to the group.

The problems of bullying and emotional dysfunction are big issues during the school days of any boy. Other more minor problems may arise, however, and these too can be helped by intelligent use of the Bach Flower Remedies. For example, some boys can miss their old, safe life at home with parents, brothers and sisters even after they have been going to school for some time – and homesickness like this is by no means confined to children at boarding school. Honeysuckle is the remedy to help boys in this state to think more of the present than the past. The remedies can also help to counter shyness (Mimulus), discouragement brought on by a failure to achieve a goal (Gentian), lethargy brought on by overwork (Olive) or mental fatigue (Hornbeam) or apathy (Wild Rose), and a thousand other situations and problems that the growing child meets as he advances towards adolescence and beyond. And Wild Oat can help an older child who has to make decisions about which subjects to study up to GCSE level and beyond, as it is the remedy to help remove uncertainty about which path to follow in life.

Broadly speaking, the emotional states experienced by children differ little from those of adults. But whereas grown men are used to the idea that they should not pay too much attention to their emotional life, and because of this are inclined to be uninformative and unresponsive when asked how they feel, boys are in almost all cases not quite so far gone. They are more likely to at least try to give straight answers to simple questions. In addition they are usually prepared to consider new ideas that older men might dismiss out of hand. All in all it can be easier to select Bach Flower Remedies for children than it is for adults.

ADOLESCENCE

For young women self-definition often involves dieting, fashion and make-up, all used by teenage girls in order to remake themselves into the people they would like to be. But, although this tactic is often contrasted with the independent ways of young men, the reality is that males do exactly the same. For some young men the quest for identity involves building up muscle, either in the gym or in the privacy of a bedroom – a fact witnessed to by the chest expanders and hand weights secreted in millions of wardrobes. For others it means adopting a persona and physical appearance drawn from music or some cult film or comic book. In these and other cases the impetus is the same: the need of the adolescent male to conform to an image of maleness, coupled with the need to find out who he really is and what he is going to be like as a man.

The would-be adult may spend months or even years trying out different types of personality and lifestyle to see which ones fit. Behaviour is understandably unpredictable at this time, and in the kaleidoscope of ideas and convictions it is no surprise that sometimes confusion sets in. There may be wild mood swings, so that one moment he is full of enthusiasm and the next in the depths of despair. Often neither condition goes on for long, but the emotions will be felt to the bone while they last, and irrespective of his feelings at any particular instant, the individual will be in a sad and destitute condition that can only be described as chronic uncertainty.

The Bach Flower Remedy for this state of indecision and constant changing is Scleranthus. Other remedies might be useful when a particular mood has actually taken over. For example, the peculiarly adolescent gloom that descends out of a clear blue sky and seems to be wholly without motive is a sure indication for the Mustard remedy. On the other hand, self-pity, sulking and resentment would need Willow.

Although Scleranthus is the remedy for indecision in general, Wild Oat may be a better choice if the problem is specifically set around an important issue, such as what religion to embrace or which career to choose, and the way ahead is confused and uncertain. People in the Wild Oat state do not usually have a problem making smaller decisions, which is one of the ways they can be told apart from Scleranthus people. Then again, other adolescents might have ideas of their own regarding what they want to do or be yet still go around asking for confirmation and advice. It is as if they do not trust their ability to make a correct choice. For them Cerato would be preferred to either Scleranthus or Wild Oat because they do know what they want and only need help to follow through their intentions.

As adolescents grow up they will be particularly conscious of the physical changes they are going through, especially as different parts of the body can develop at different rates. It is usual, for example, for the legs and arms to grow before the trunk, and it is this that leads to the typically gawky appearance of some teenage boys. Boys may also be embarrassed by late sexual development and the lingering appearance of 'bum fluff' when their friends are already shaving. This sort of unhappiness with one's appearance can be a source of despair or self-hatred. Gorse would be the remedy for the first, Crab Apple for the second.

In some – fortunately rare – cases the confusions and anxieties of adolescence get so bad that teenagers consider taking their own lives. Once more, adolescent suicides are far more likely to be male than female. Sometimes there is some deep underlying reason for suicidal thoughts, such as family breakdown or a very low self-image. But at other times the teeming emotions of the adolescent can leave him open to an apparently trivial upset, and failing an exam or a relatively minor medical problem can be taken completely out of proportion. In any case, talk of suicide should always be taken seriously. Never think that it is just attention-seeking and be tempted to ignore it. Neither should you dismiss a suicide attempt as just a cry for help, because this particular cry for help might be the last cry the victim ever utters. Cherry Plum is the remedy to help alleviate suicidal thoughts and violent thoughts of all kinds, and professional help should also be sought as a matter of urgency.

You might also consider getting professional help faced with other extremes of behaviour. Risk-taking is common in the teenage years, and one of the commonest examples of the phenomenon is experimenting with drugs, for example:

- Tobacco
- Cannabis
- Ecstasy
- Alcohol
- Heroin
- Crack cocaine

Males are more prone to this behaviour, perhaps because the prevailing male mystique demands that they show their peers how well they can handle danger and risk.

Particular drugs might be especially popular among specific types of adolescent. For example, those who are shy and find social events difficult might turn to alcohol because of its effects on inhibition or find the ability to talk to people by taking amphetamines. Other drugs, especially ecstasy, are associated with lifestyles and types of music. The young man who wants to get into that lifestyle is pretty much forced to take the drug as part of the package.

When dealing with drug abuse it is essential to start by telling the truth. As I tried to demonstrate in the list a few paragraphs back, some of the drugs that the adult world accepts and promotes are as risky and dangerous as illegal ones. If you lecture a teenager about his once-a-week cannabis cigarette while you are smoking your twentieth cigarette of the day you are inviting ridicule. Just as bad is the pretence that taking drugs will inevitably lead to sickness, social breakdown and death. Teenagers look at their healthy, socially active and lively drug-taking friends and believe what they see rather than what society tells them. Be honest and you might find out more about the roots of the drug-taking. Once you have done this you will be in a better position to decide what remedies might help. For example, the shy alcohol drinker might benefit from

Mimulus. A lack of confidence in social situations might also be helped with Larch. And Wild Rose might help where apathy about life, work and relationships left the person an easy prey to drug-induced stupor.

When risk-taking goes too far it shades into criminal activity, such as arson, vandalism, theft and even violence against others. Often the roots of this are found in peer-group pressure, which might be resisted more successfully with the help of Walnut. Resentment can also be a cause, whether against one's family, schoolteachers or society as a whole. Willow is the remedy for such self-pitying, negative emotions. Other youths are motivated by hatred of those who are more successful, or richer, better-looking or whatever, and in these cases Holly would be the remedy to choose. Beech could be given to help those who lack tolerance of other people and other ways of life. Those teenagers who indulge in racist abuse and violence would be obvious cases for treatment with Beech. But criminal behaviour could also be an expression of hopelessness at, for example, a lack of employment opportunities or family breakdown. Gorse or Sweet Chestnut could be given to counteract such feelings, depending on their strength and exact nature. Those who repeatedly fall back into their delinquent behaviour despite being helped to stop over and over again might need Chestnut Bud to help them learn and move on.

The same extremes of reaction can be seen in those adolescents who seek not to destroy but to change for the better. They are the teenage idealists and the would-be revolutionaries. They dislike and have no hesitation in denouncing what they see as hypocrisy and unnecessary compromise, especially in their parents. Their impatience with the way things are and with older people who support the status quo might be tempered with Impatiens. There is a Beech element of intolerance as well. Those teenagers who become self-righteous and arrogant about their own beliefs might be softened by this remedy. Otherwise, Vervain is the remedy for the kind of commitment and enthusiasm that can lead to fanaticism and leave the highly-strung adolescent exhausted and unable to switch off.

In all these cases the treatment aim is to help the fiery adolescent see other sides of questions and understand opposing points of view, even if he does not come to share them. It is not to make the individual lose his idealism. There is full-blooded beauty in idealism when it serves natural justice and honour. Jaded adults could learn a great deal from the simplicity, honesty and commitment with which adolescents support their causes.

EXAMINATIONS

The competitive world of school is punctuated by the even more intense competition of examinations. At first exams might seem unimportant to most boys, but as they get older so exam results have a more direct impact, not just on prestige and self-image but on earning potential and the immediate future. When you consider that going to university or starting a career may depend on two and a half hours in an exam room, it is no surprise that exam nerves are very common.

Whatever the sufferers may think, there is no relationship between ability and anxiety. Even the best students can suffer from exam nerves, and the people who sail through their examinations with total confidence do not always do as well as they thought they would. Nevertheless extreme nerves can affect performance and will certainly make life pretty unpleasant while they last, so it is fortunate that there are a number of tried and tested techniques that can help prepare for exams and overcome nerves. And the Bach Flower Remedies can help as well, of course.

In all likelihood the commonest anti-exam remedy in the Bach repertory is Rescue Remedy. It is ready to hand when needed and it contains remedies calculated to help people faced with a crisis, such as the remedies for terror (Rock Rose), shock (Star of Bethlehem) and agitation (Impatiens). Larch too has a good reputation as a specific against exam nerves, since it is the remedy to restore confidence. Some people take a bottle of one or other of these remedies into the examination room along with their pens and pencils. This is a good idea and worth adopting, but it doesn't alter the fact that the best time to start combatting nerves is well before the exam itself starts.

By planning his revision before he actually starts work and then sticking to his plan, the ideal student will at least approach the coming ordeal with a certain amount of confidence. A revision plan should include clear and achievable objectives, each one plainly marked with a date by which it should have been done. It is much easier to work to a timetable that covers French regular verbs by Wednesday, irregular verbs by Friday and the conditional tense by Sunday afternoon than it is to try to "do" French sometime next week. The plan should also include time for rest and relaxation, preferably built in as a reward for a task completed thoroughly and on time. Finally, it is a good idea to start revising a subject by picking the topic that is most interesting, or failing that the one that is easiest. This will help get the whole revision process off to a flying start.

An essential technique that many students forget when they start to revise is this: remember to think. It sounds obvious, but people find it all too easy to read notes in a mechanical way so that by the time they get to page 20 they haven't got the least idea what was on page 19, let alone page one. The best way to avoid this is to make additional notes while reading. This doesn't mean copying things out word for word as they appear in the original notes, but rather paraphrasing, a process which forces the mind to think through the subject one more time. It is also a good idea to ask questions all the time, such as: would so-and-so agree with this point? What other points of view could be put across? Are there exceptions to this rule? The student who questions the things he reads will remember far more than the one who tries to learn words in a book off by heart.

Ideally the night before the exam the candidate will be so well prepared that he will be able to relax, watch a little television or read a novel and get a good night's sleep. Even if he is not quite up to this he should not plan on staying up all night engaged in last-minute revision as this is bound to be counter-productive. His time would be better spent making sure he has all the pens and other equipment he will need for the next day. If he does want a last check of his notes he should only look over the topics that he has already revised – this is not a good time to try to learn a new subject.

On the day of the exam the ideal is to arrive in plenty of time.

But if some unforeseen event causes you to arrive late it is important not to panic – take some Rescue Remedy instead and think things through calmly. The time allowed for each exam question can be adjusted so that the required number of questions can be at least attempted. This is a tactic that is far more likely to lead to a pass than answering two questions fully when the examiners asked for three. And it is still a good idea, irrespective of how late you arrived, to try to leave at least ten minutes at the end of the exam so that there is time to read through the written answers and correct any obvious factual or grammatical errors.

Of course few people in practice are able to live up to this ideal plan without some help. If you are one of them, there are a number of ways of helping yourself. First of all you need to fight against any tendency you might feel to give up without a struggle. Maybe you have found the subject harder than you expected and are convinced you will fail; or maybe you have done badly at exams in the past and think of yourself as one of those people who cannot do exams. A number of the Bach Flower Remedies might help in this instance: Larch for the lack of confidence; Gentian for the discouragement that you feel; Chestnut Bud if the previous exam failures can be traced to the same bad practice on your part. Maybe it is the sheer importance of the exam that is frightening you, and the thought of what a failure might mean to your future career. Mimulus is the remedy for a named fear, and could certainly help in this case. But you might also consider Gentian, which might help you to look beyond the difficulties and so approach the challenge in a more optimistic frame of mind, and Larch again, which should help strengthen not only your faith in your ability but also give you the courage needed to cope with success or failure. After all, failing an exam is not the end of life or ambition, and the history books are full of famous, creative and successful men who started their careers by failing their exams.

If the hard work of revision has left you tired and drained, Olive is the remedy to restore strength. That other form of tiredness, when you wake up after a good night's sleep full of weariness and unable to take up your books again, would be helped by Hornbeam. This is a mental rather than a physical tiredness and should soon go once you summon the resolve to start work again. And if you continue to work on despite your tiredness, when you really ought to rest, then Oak, Rock Water or Vervain might be indicated: the first if you plod on remorselessly; the second if you force yourself to do too much out of a misguided sense of self-discipline; the last if pure enthusiasm and mental energy are to blame.

If you are anxious before or during the exam there are a great many other techniques you can use to help you. David Acres' helpful book *How to Pass Exams Without Anxiety* mentions many of them, including:

- Talking positively to yourself (negative thoughts could be helped by Gentian, Larch, Willow or Heather – or many other remedies – depending on the exact nature of the mental state being addressed).
- Thinking about and preparing for anxiety-causing situations before they arise (Mimulus is the remedy for known fears; Aspen for vague, groundless anxiety and Rock Rose the specific against terror).
- Thinking about the next task you need to complete rather than some vague end result way off in the future (Clematis would help if this is a tendency you have).
- Thinking about the present rather than the past (Honeysuckle).
- Concentrating on the things you can change rather than worrying over factors outside your control (White Chestnut is the remedy for uncontrolled and unwanted thoughts).
- Learning relaxation techniques (if you have trouble relaxing because you are too fired up, Vervain could be the remedy to help).
- Stopping worrying thoughts (White Chestnut again, or Agrimony if you conceal your worries behind a smile).
- Developing a balanced lifestyle (many remedies can help here, depending on the kind of person you are; Scleranthus in particular helps if you are subject to mood swings).

As the indications in brackets suggest, many of the Bach Flower Remedies can be directly related to David Acres' suggestions.

So far the problems discussed in relation to exams apply as much to girls as to boys. But the kind of machismo which deliberately courts failure is far more common among male than among female students. Being 'one of the boys' implies not taking too much trouble over study and not worrying unduly about academic matters. In their desire not to be thought lacking in manly qualities adolescent boys are particularly inclined to make a virtue of failure. At least it proves that they are independent and not frightened of what their parents or teachers will say. The fact that their conformity to the cult of machismo is itself rooted in fear – the fear of seeming different from the people in their gang – is of course largely unnoticed.

Mimulus is the remedy to deal with fears like this, that can be named and analysed, but other remedies might be useful as well as or instead of Mimulus. For example, Walnut is the link-breaking remedy that helps free people from the unwanted influence of ideas and attitudes that are holding them back from success. Centaury might be a help to those who have a tendency to follow other people's bad examples and find it hard to stand up for their own principles, and Wild Rose could be given if an affected apathy and fatalism has become a habit.

Inevitably the day will come when the examinations are long over and the results arrive. If everything has passed off well then there will be excited preparations for college, university or the start of working life. Apprehension and nerves go along with these, of course, and can be treated in the usual way.

Things are more serious if the results are not all that had been hoped. In this case it is normal to feel discouraged (Gentian) and perhaps inclined to throw in the towel without trying again (Gorse). Guilt and useless regret are also common: if only the failed student had worked harder, gone to more classes or started revising earlier then maybe things would have been different. Even the devil-may-care may start to fret over what their teachers and parents will think of their performance, and may blame themselves for letting others down. Pine is the remedy for guilt and Honeysuckle deals with regrets over one's past actions. For those who are feeling sorry for themselves or resentful that other people have done better than they have, Willow should be chosen. Rock Water can help people who feel they have failed to live up to their own high standards, and Heather is for those who lose all sense of proportion and see their own often rather minor failures as bigger and more important than anyone else's. Finally, people who genuinely feel that the failure has destroyed their future could try Sweet Chestnut, which is the remedy for ultimate despair and anguish. It is also a good idea to talk to someone, because this is a state of mind that may need extra help.

The aim of using the Bach Flower Remedies at this time is of course to help the sufferer see that failing one (or all) his exams is not the end of things, only the opening of new and different opportunities. He may be able to retake the exams later in the year, or perhaps he can change tack entirely and do something entirely different and perhaps more worthwhile with his life. What he needs to do is investigate the alternatives as soon as possible, and with the help of the Bach Flower Remedies he should, with luck, be able to start doing that sooner rather than later.

CHAPTER 2

SEX

FIRST STEPS WITH SEX

During puberty and adolescence boys become more interested in sexuality and in potential sexual partners, and sex is thought about more than most would care to admit. But even if they are experts in the mechanics of the sex act few young men have any idea how to get close to girls, while for others there is added confusion in the suspicion that they might not be attracted to girls at all, but to other males. Most (probably all) young men, whatever their orientation, turn to masturbation as a quick way of obtaining sexual satisfaction without having to deal with the problems that a full sexual partnership would inevitably bring.

Despite its wholly negative connotations in male company – the word 'wanker' is a common term of abuse – just about every boy starts to masturbate somewhere between the ages of ten and sixteen, and many men go on masturbating for the rest of their lives. There is nothing wrong with this, of course. Whatever the threats of folk wisdom masturbation does not cause blindness, madness or spots. But the taboos surrounding the subject and the fear of being found out lead to all kinds of psychological problems. Even today many boys go through agonies thinking they are the only ones doing this terrible thing.

Groundless guilt is of course one very common reaction, and Pine would be the remedy to ease this. Mimulus can be tried for anyone who naively believes that masturbation will do him some harm and so is fearful of the consequences if he goes on. Where there is a vague feeling of insecurity and anxiety associated with the practice, the same superstitious beliefs might have been repressed so that there seems no specific reason for them. Aspen would be the remedy for this shifting kind of fear.

With many men masturbation continues even after full inter-course has been started. The reasons for feeling guilty might be slightly different now. It can be seen as a rejection of one's sexual partner since if sex were being thoroughly enjoyed there would be no need to masturbate. Other men assume that continuing to masturbate when there is no obvious need to is a sign of some kind of moral weakness, or evidence of a lack of maturity. Again, there is simply no evidence that masturbation at any stage of life does any harm or interferes with normal sex and consequently there is no reason to be ashamed or guilty about doing it.

The first experience of non-masturbatory sex can itself cause emotional problems. First of all it can all too easily be an immense disappointment, even a humiliation, especially where both partners are inexperienced. If they care for each other this is less likely to matter. But if – as so often happens – sex is simply the next step that a couple feel they are expected to take or a chance encounter based on curiosity and opportunity rather than emotional need then the results can be very upsetting.

Sometimes the experience can be so bad that Star of Bethlehem, the remedy for shock, or Rescue Remedy may be needed. Crab Apple would be the remedy to select where a clumsy and insensitive encounter leaves the man or his partner feeling dirty and disgusted at their own sexuality. These feelings are rare, however, and most negative reactions to the first time are confined to disappointment and despondency (Gentian), self-reproach and guilt (Pine), and anxiety over the risk of pregnancy, catching a sexually transmitted diseases, or, more mundanely, of one's parents finding out. Mimulus is the remedy for these known fears.

Failing to get to the first time also brings problems. Resentment may follow against others who seem to be doing so much better: Willow is the remedy for this emotion. If the virginal state goes on even longer the young man may begin to lose his confidence and start to believe that he will never be a success or manage to attract a partner. Larch is the remedy in this case to give him back his confidence. Of the other types of personality Dr Bach identified, Water Violet people in particular may find difficulty getting to know potential partners since their natural quietness and reserve can make them appear aloof and uninterested in others. The remedy can help them to relax and engage more in society, although only of course when they want to.

Such is the pressure in our society to be seen to be sexually active that there is great temptation among young men to conceal their virginity when it becomes embarrassing to them. If it spares their blushes, they are happy to laugh and joke about fictional partners. Agrimony might be an appropriate remedy if the person indulging in this behaviour was feeling, and hiding, genuine pain over his inability to find a mate.

The virgin's struggle is as nothing to the young homosexual's. Despite the many years of political struggle by advocates of gay rights there is no doubt that society as a whole is far less tolerant of homosexuality than it might be. All too many people profess their acceptance of gays while at the same time abhorring any open sign of affection between lovers of the same sex and insisting that the whole thing should be carried on in secret, like any other crime. This is all the stranger as study after study has shown that it is quite common for otherwise heterosexual men to be attracted to their own sex for a time in adolescence. Presumably many of the strongest critics of homosexuality are among those who have experienced just such a phase, and are now busily repressing it or explaining it to themselves in more neutral terms.

The need to hide one's sexuality leads to a life full of unnecessary deceit, fear and uncertainty for the male homosexual. It is all the worse as so much of his upbringing will have instilled in him the need to be a real man after the hairy-handed heterosexual model, so that the discovery that he is something other can come as a bitter and terrifying blow. The straight world would do well to reflect upon the courage needed to be yourself when the rest of the world assumes and insists that you are something quite different.

The Bach Flower Remedies will not of course cure homosexuals of their homosexuality. They could hardly begin to do so as sexuality is not a state of illness or wellness but an expression of what you are. As the whole philosophy of the remedies is to help people live in accordance with their own personalities and wishes, the treatment goal in the case of homosexuals is to help them retain their balance and go their own ways free of guilt, pain and negative emotions of any kind.

Among the remedies that might help are Scleranthus, Cerato, Walnut, Mimulus, Red Chestnut, Pine and Gentian:

- Scleranthus is for doubt, hesitation and uncertainty when the person finds that doubt about his sexuality seems to paralyse his ability to make any decisions.
- Cerato is for those who know their own hearts but lack the conviction to go their own way and distrust their own conclusions. Consequently they may ask other people for advice all the time and end up more confused than ever.
- Walnut is of course the link-breaker. It can help to overcome past ties and habits that make the birth of an emerging sexuality more problematic than it needs to be.
- Mimulus is for those who are scared of the effect their sexuality will have when it is known about. They may fear losing their friends, the reaction of parents and possible repercussions due to homophobic attitudes held by employers, teachers and other people in authority. For all these fears Mimulus would be indicated.
- Where the fear is felt on behalf of others, so that the possible effect that a declaration might have on the happiness of loved ones is the problem, then Red Chestnut would be preferred.
- Pine is for feelings of guilt at hurting other people or disappointing expectations.
- Gentian would be a help to those men whose plans to come out are frustrated by some setback which leaves them doubting how to pick up the pieces again.

If all the above sounds too negative it should be stressed that for the vast majority of men the discovery of sex is an exciting and overwhelmingly pleasurable experience, whatever their sexual orientation or the date at which the discovery starts. The Bach Flower Remedies are always there to help, but there should be no question of looking for problems where none in fact exist.

CONTRACEPTION

Contraceptives can be divided into two groups according to who generally takes responsibility for them. The first and largest group is made up of precautions taken mainly or wholly by women. They are listed here, with approximate failure rates shown in brackets. The failure rate is defined as the percentage of women who will become pregnant in a year if they rely on a particular method.

- Coil (1.5%)
- Diaphragm (2%)
- Female condom (7%)
- Morning-after pill (4%)
- Pill (0.3 to 1.5% depending on type)
- Rhythm method (up to 15%)
- Spermicidal gel (12%)
- Sterilisation (0.13%)

That leaves the following three methods which are usually the responsibility of the male partner.

- Condoms (4%)
- Vasectomy (0.02%)
- Withdrawal (35%)

In a sense this is an artificial distinction, since in an ideal world couples would make the choice of contraceptive together and after carefully weighing up all the factors. But as this book is concerned with men and their reactions to life situations this is not really the place to discuss those forms of contraception that we have classed as female. In this part of the book, then, we will concentrate on the last three methods since they more directly affect the male.

Of the three, vasectomy is overwhelmingly the surest method if one looks purely and simply at the prevention of pregnancy. In practice, though, it is only available to older men who can satisfy doctors that they have all the children they are ever going to want. Although the operation to sever the tube that carries sperm from the testes can in some cases be reversed, the failure rate for such reversals is high. Men who are considering a vasectomy and having difficulty deciding whether to go ahead with it or not could try Scleranthus to help them to see things more clearly. The motives and hesitations of people in this position will come under examination long before the operation can go ahead.

Vasectomy itself is a straightforward procedure and unless there is some medical complication it will usually be carried out under local anaesthetic and without the need for a stay in hospital. The ability to have an erection, achieve orgasm and ejaculate will not be impaired, and the vast majority of men say that their sex-lives improve after the operation. A very small proportion (around 2%) say the opposite, and those who are unlucky enough to number themselves in this percentage might need to turn to the Bach Flower Remedies to correct what is probably a psychological impediment rather than a physical one.

Withdrawal is the least satisfactory method of contraception from any point of view. However careful a man is to pull his penis out of his partner before he climaxes he can never be sure that sperm has not already entered her. This is because small amounts of semen leak from the penis during intercourse, so that withdrawal may be too late however early in intercourse it takes place. In addition there is the risk of bad timing. It is not always that easy to pace a climax, and in the heat of the moment the temptation to keep going for just a half second more may be too much to resist. The fact that the most fertile gush of semen is the first one makes any delay doubly dangerous. In addition, although the talk of physical and mental problems caused by coitus interruptus is almost certainly without foundation, withdrawal may still give the end of love-making a rushed and artificial feel and it provides no defence against sexually-transmitted disease.

For most men then the only form of contraception that they normally have direct contact with is the condom. Dating from the time of the Roman empire, the humble prophylactic is actually enjoying something of a renaissance at the moment with television, jeans manufacturers, record companies and youth magazines all doing their best to make it popular and trendy. The reason for all these efforts is of course AIDS and the HIV virus that causes it.

Condoms are the only form of contraception to offer limited protection against the transmission of HIV, a degree of safety which is improved when condoms are used in conjunction with a spermicidal gel such as Nonoxynol 9, which helps kill the virus if it is present.

Before the adverts and the press campaigns the condom had been for many years the least popular contraceptive device among men. Feminists might say that this was because it was the only one that inconvenienced men instead of women, and it would be hard to argue with this analysis. But in addition it has to be said that there is nothing inherently sensual or aesthetically pleasing or romantic about opening an aluminium package and unrolling a piece of rubber in the middle of an otherwise passionate embrace. What's more there is a slight but noticeable loss of sensation in the penis. It isn't even as reliable as other 'approved' forms of contraception such as the pill, the coil and the diaphragm.

Nevertheless, AIDS alone means that anyone who is in anything other than a strictly monogamous, long-term and stable relationship should be using condoms. Men who refuse to wear them are behaving very stupidly and putting themselves and their partners at risk. And as much of the failure rate of condoms can be traced to breakages and other preventable accidents it's as well to learn how to use them correctly. Here then are the do's and don'ts of condom use:

- DO use a condom coated with Nonoxynol 9 spermicidal gel.
- DO squeeze the air out of the teat at the top of the condom before you put it on – if you don't the condom is more likely to break.
- DO use regular or heavyweight condoms instead of very thin ones – they offer better protection.
- DO put the condom on as soon as you have an erection, and in any case before you get anywhere near penetration.
- DO hold onto the bottom of the condom when you withdraw from your lover to prevent leakage.
- DON'T use a condom if the foil wrapping is damaged or the condom is past its 'use by' date.

- DON'T scratch or tear condoms with fingernails, teeth etc.
- DON'T use massage oils or other lubricants with condoms unless they are specifically designed for the purpose (some oils weaken the rubber and make breakage more likely).
- DON'T use the same condom more than once.

Some men seem able to use condoms for years and years without ever learning these simple rules, even though many of them can be found printed in every packet of condoms sold. Consequently they enjoy – if that's the word – an unacceptably high failure rate. Despite repeated experiment they can't seem to learn that putting condoms on incorrectly makes them burst and gives no protection to anyone. If this sounds like you, add two drops of Chestnut Bud to a treatment bottle and try a little harder next time.

SEXUALLY-TRANSMITTED DISEASES

Sexually-transmitted diseases (or STD's) are diseases that happen to be transmitted through sexual intercourse. That's all they are. But the fact that they are associated with sex and in particular with casual or promiscuous sex has invested them with a peculiar significance. If you catch 'flu or yellow fever you will feel sorry for yourself; if you catch a sexually-transmitted disease you will probably feel ashamed of yourself as well.

Partly as a response to the emotional impact of STD's special anonymous clinics have been set up in hospitals around the country. People who are reluctant to take their symptoms to their family doctor can go to the clinics and receive free, non-judgmental diagnosis, counselling and treatment.

It is essential that people who think they might be suffering from a sexually-transmitted disease get proper medical help as soon as possible. There are ten main STD's, all of which can affect both men and women, although they are more or less common according to gender and often the symptoms are markedly different. Most conditions are curable and all can be alleviated with the latest treatment. The ten are:

AIDS

Acquired Immune Deficiency Syndrome is the latest and most serious of STD's. It is caused by HIV (Human Immunodeficiency Virus), a virus that is passed from person to person in body fluids such as semen and blood. The first real signs that a person has been infected with HIV can come up to 10 years after infection with the development of either full-blown AIDS, characterised by extreme weight loss and a variety of serious illnesses including various cancers and pneumonia, or AIDS-Related Complex, which has various symptoms including weight loss, tiredness and night sweats. Up until the appearance of definite symptoms sufferers may have no knowledge that they have been infected, and this long latent period obviously makes it harder to prevent the spread of the disease. AIDS is eventually fatal in almost all cases and there is no known cure, although some treatments are believed to slow down the onset of the disease, and the secondary infections that go along with it can be treated in the normal way.

In Britain AIDS is commonest in male homosexuals, where a relatively promiscuous lifestyle and the increased risk associated with anal sex helped it take a hold early on. In many other parts of the world including Asia and Africa heterosexual men and women make up the vast majority of cases.

Despite the rash of scare stories in the mid eighties HIV is not transmitted through sitting on toilet seats, sharing cups or kissing. Unprotected sex (i.e. sex without a condom), anal intercourse, and infection by means of dirty hypodermic syringes and unscreened blood products are the main infection routes.

CANDIDIASIS

Candidiasis is better known by the common name thrush. It is a fungal infection that can cause inflammation, but it is easily treated and not a threat to general health. Many men can be infected and never know about it unless their partners develop symptoms.

CHANCROID

This disease causes painful, ulcerous pimples to appear on the penis around a week after intercourse. It is very rare in Britain but is curable provided medical advice is sought.

GENITAL HERPES

Before AIDS came along genital herpes was the subject of a number of scare stories in the British press, mostly hinging on the word 'incurable'. In fact genital herpes is a variation on the common cold sore and in men at least is usually little more than an inconvenience. The symptoms for infected women are more severe. Like cold sores, people who have been infected are always liable to repeat attacks since the herpes virus lies dormant in the body until stress or illness gives it an opportunity to attack again. There are treatments available that can help cure an attack very quickly, but infected men should certainly abstain from sexual intercourse until the ulcers have entirely disappeared as they are very infectious.

GENITAL WARTS

Genital warts are not dangerous to men, but in women are linked to cervical cancer. Because of this both partners should abstain from sex and seek treatment if they suspect that one or both have been infected – although in practice this can be difficult to do since the warts can be practically invisible to the naked eye. Where they are visible they are small and clustered, usually around the foreskin.

Sometimes people are tempted to treat genital warts themselves using commercial products designed for removing ordinary warts from other areas of the body. This is dangerous, and should not be attempted under any circumstances.

GONORRHOEA

Gonorrhoea is one of the world's most common infectious diseases, second only to measles. The symptoms are a discharge from the penis and pain on passing water, usually starting between 3 and 10 days after intercourse. The treatment is by antibiotics and is fairly routine, but it is important to get help early on because, if left, the infection may spread and male victims can be left sterile. Symptoms may disappear for a while, but if the infection is not treated it will not go away by itself, so anyone who thinks he might be infected should seek advice as soon as possible.

HEPATITIS B

This is an infection of the liver caused by a virus that is passed on through sexual intercourse or contact with infected blood, much as the HIV virus is. The classic symptoms of Hepatitis B are yellowing skin and eyes caused by jaundice, fatigue and nausea – but some people do not have any of these symptoms, making it hard to prevent infection from spreading. Most people are able to recover completely after a period of rest and perhaps hospitalization, but a large minority suffer permanent liver damage.

NON-GONOCOCCAL URETHRITIS (NGU)

NGU is more common in men than in women. The symptoms at first are similar to those of gonorrhoea, with a discharge from the penis and pain in the urethra when urinating. These symptoms appear within one to four weeks after intercourse. The treatment is complete sexual abstinence coupled with doses of antibiotic – and it is essential to get treatment because if nothing is done the infection will spread and may cause many kinds of illnesses including a recurrent and potentially disfiguring form of arthritis.

SYPHILIS

Fortunately syphilis is much rarer than it once was, and is no longer a feared killer since it can be completely cured with penicillin – as long as it is caught early enough. The first sign to look for is a pimple on the penis which appears about three weeks after intercourse. This develops into a painless, hardened ulcer which takes several weeks to fade, usually leaving a scar. This stage is known as primary syphilis and if treatment is sought now it is relatively easy to effect a cure.

Secondary syphilis occurs around 6 weeks after the initial infection, when a pinkish rash develops on the body and spreads to the face. At the same time the sufferer may feel unwell, with headaches and a sore throat. Sometimes flattened ulcers appear in the mouth or around the genitals. Eventually these symptoms fade, but if the disease remains untreated tertiary syphilis eventually occurs, usually many years later. This final stage is characterised by mental decay and severe disorders of the heart, bone and skin.

TRICHOMONIASIS

This is similar to candidiasis, but is caused by an animal called a flagellate rather than a fungus. Usually the only way a man can tell he might have trichomoniasis is when his partner is diagnosed, at which time they will both be treated with a week-long course of tablets.

Probably the only completely sure way not to get a sexually-transmitted disease is not to have sex. Failing that, sticking to a monogamous relationship is almost as good. The third option – realistically the only option for a very large number of people – is to take precautions. These are all fairly obvious: restrict the number of sexual partners; never make love without wearing a condom; look for obvious signs of infection in a new partner; and go to the doctor at once if there is any reason to fear an infection.

The Bach Flower Remedies are not designed to treat physical complaints like these, and are not a replacement for medical attention. What they can do is help to remove the emotional baggage that goes along with this whole subject, leaving people free to make balanced and informed choices about who they sleep with and when to go for medical advice. For example:

- If someone is frightened that he might have a sexually-transmitted disease Mimulus can help to calm the fear so that he can think rationally about what to do next.
- The man who is unsure whether to see the doctor or not may need Scleranthus to help him to reach a decision and act on it.
- People who are inclined to shrug their shoulders and accept their symptoms as beyond their control can be helped with Wild Rose.
- Useless worrying thoughts while waiting for test results would need White Chestnut.

Where someone has gone to the doctor and his fears have proved well-founded the remedies are there to help again. Feelings of guilt would call for Pine. Disgust at one's physical state would call for Crab Apple, and resentment against the person from whom the infection was contracted would be helped with Willow. Someone who has contracted many STD's might learn from Chestnut Bud not to repeat the same mistake next time he is offered unsafe sex.

Of all the diseases mentioned earlier in this section only two are incurable and of those only one is serious and potentially fatal. If you have had the misfortune to be diagnosed as HIV-positive you will need all the support and friendship that you can get. There are numerous charities and other organisations who go some way to provide this kind of help, but despite their efforts and your own attempts to be strong and come to terms with your condition there are bound to be times when you will feel depressed and alone.

There are no miracle cures, unfortunately, but you are not helpless. Many doctors from all kinds of different traditions now accept that a positive mental outlook is one of the most important weapons you have in the fight against HIV and AIDS. It is important to love yourself, to be yourself, and to stay on an even keel, and in all these things the remedies can have a role to play. To give just a few examples:

- Star of Bethlehem can help deal with the great shock of the diagnosis.
- Rock Rose is for the terror that might stop you from thinking rationally about your situation.
- Gorse would be indicated if you felt hopeless despair at your situation.
- Sweet Chestnut would be for the even blacker moments when there seemed to be no future of any type and no possible way forward.
- If you struggle to go on as normal, going to work and coming home like everyone else, but feel your strength and perseverance about to crack, Oak is your type remedy and can help restore your normal courage.
- Wild Rose is for moments of complete apathy, when you don't see any purpose or reason to go on getting out of bed. It may help to reawaken your sense of purpose and interest in life.

These are examples, not prescriptions. Your actual reactions to such an overwhelming event will depend very much on your personality, and in this as in all matters the Bach system is clear: if a positive outcome is to be achieved it is the person who must be considered first, not the disease.

PROBLEMS WITH SEX

Men set great store by their sexual prowess, and being able to perform well in bed is intimately bound up with male notions of success in love and relationships. Consequently any suggestion of impotence can be very traumatic, especially as many men seem to think that the ability to achieve penetration is the sole factor that separates a good performance from a bad one. The stress men lay on the mechanics of sex is all the more unfortunate because most men will suffer temporary mechanical breakdown at some time in their lives.

Impotence – the inability to achieve or maintain an erection – can have any of several root causes. A heavy night's drinking is well-known as a cause of 'brewer's droop', but overwork, tiredness and emotional problems can all have as great an impact. The fact that impotence is often entirely psychological is shown by the fact that men recovering from a heart attack often suffer a period of impotence because they are frightened that intercourse will cause a further attack. In older men age might be a factor: the angle of erection declines steadily from the early twenties, and later on less testosterone is produced. The start of a new relationship may also be a testing time. While some men find the novelty exciting, others find their anxiety levels increase because they want to perform well but aren't sure what the other person will expect, and this increased anxiety can make it difficult to get or maintain an erection. The answer to all these problems is of course to relax and get to know one's partner better. Prolonged foreplay will achieve both these goals at once and will in itself make sex enjoyable whether or not penetration takes place.

Other possible physical causes of impotence, besides alcohol, include the effects of cannabis, some anti-depressants, and drugs taken against ulcers, high blood pressure and diabetes. If the problem continues it is a good idea to seek medical help. Even if the cause is psychological the doctor will be able to help in most cases, or will be able to refer the problem on to someone else better qualified.

A much rarer problem than impotence is premature ejaculation. This is where ejaculation takes place during foreplay or very early on in intercourse. As with impotence, anxiety is one of the main causes, and again it is no surprise that, as a problem, it is particularly associated with new sexual partners.

Occasionally a man simply loses interest in sex. This can happen after prolonged illness or when he is under stress at work, or overtired, or when his relationship with his partner is going through a bad patch. For some men saying they are not interested in sex any more may be a way of covering anxiety about impotence or other fears about performance. It is important if at all possible that men in this position share fears like these with their partners. If a problem within the relationship is causing the loss of libido then that is the problem that has to be solved before anything else.

The role of the Bach Flower Remedies in all these conditions is to treat the emotional negativity that can lie concealed under the surface of the apparent symptoms. They cannot replace medication for specifically physical problems, of course, but they may help to maintain a positive frame of mind and promote relaxation. Where the root of the problem is emotional, this may be all that is required for things to improve.

As always the precise selection of remedies will depend on the individual man's personality and emotional state, but the following indications are among the most common:

- There might be some shock when the problem is first noticed, and for this Star of Bethlehem is the remedy to choose.
- Feelings of disgust or distaste for sex and for the body in general, whether prior to or subsequent to the problem, could be helped with Crab Apple. This is the cleansing remedy, and will also help those people whose problems with sex are based on negative feelings about their own appearance, and those who suffer from an exaggerated fear of sexually-transmitted disease.

- Some men, especially those who are normally very controlled and repressed, may be afraid to unbend and relax enough to begin enjoying sex. Rock Water is the remedy for such types.
- For other specific fears and anxieties the first remedy to look into would be Mimulus.
- Those men who have lost confidence in their ability to make love successfully might try Larch.
- Where boredom is the problem Wild Rose might help, or Chestnut Bud to get the sufferer out of the repetitive cycle of behaviour that has got him into a rut.
- Hornbeam is the remedy to try where the thought of sex is wearisome but the appetite returns as soon as foreplay begins.
- For physical tiredness Oak, Elm or Vervain might be indicated depending on the type of person being treated and his current circumstances.
- Where there is physical tiredness without any particular negative mental states being to blame then Olive is the natural choice to restore lost vigour.

Worrying about sexual problems can be particularly counter-productive, not only failing to find answers but making things even worse. For constant worriers who find it hard to concentrate on anything else White Chestnut is the remedy to select. Agrimony is the remedy for worries that surface at quiet moments in the day but are mostly pushed to the back of the mind by extrovert behaviour. If someone experiences a very minor problem but allows it to get out of proportion, perhaps becoming tearful and inflicting his self-obsessed worries on other people at inappropriate moments, then Heather would be the remedy to choose.

It should be stressed again that the remedies can be used in a complementary way with problems like these. Help is available from general practitioners or, for those who prefer to be more anonymous, from clinics and professional sex therapists. Anyone who experiences any long-lasting or severe bout of impotence, or any other sexual dysfunction, is strongly advised to seek such help. And a doctor should always be consulted if a man is suffering from pain in his penis after making love. The cause could be as simple as an allergy to a make of condom or to a gel or pessary being used by his partner, but he might also be suffering from an infection that may need treatment.

It is especially important to see a doctor if erections themselves are painful or the glans of the penis is inflamed or swollen. The first symptom could indicate a disorder called priapism, and the second is probably evidence that the individual is suffering from an infection called balanitis. Both of these conditions should be treated as soon as possible by a qualified medical practitioner.

TOWARDS A FULFILLING SEX LIFE

Men will go a long way and do the strangest things in order to be more attractive to women and better in bed. They will spend hours lifting weights to sculpt the perfect body. They will try to delay orgasm by thinking about cricket scores or the holes in their socks. Some of them will even pay a small fortune to undergo painful and potentially hazardous surgery aimed at increasing the size of their penises. They'll do anything, it seems, except listen to what their partners actually want.

Study after study has shown that penis size comes very low on the list of desirable qualities. A woman's vagina only ever opens enough to allow entry so that regardless of size the actual contact between penis and vagina will be the same. Heavily-muscled bodies are actually a turn-off to most women, who prefer their men to be slim rather than muscle-bound. As for thinking about cricket and holed socks – imagine how you would feel if your partner spent your most intimate shared moments considering what to wear to work next day or recapping the plot of last night's soap opera. What women actually want was indicated by the Hite Report in the mid 1970s. They want more affection – cuddles, hugs and embraces – and more emotional engagement by men. They want to be treated as sexual and emotional equals rather than aids to masturbation. They want good sex, of course, but this does not necessarily equate with penetration.

This last point is particularly interesting. A lot of men seem to believe that everything in sex is designed simply to facilitate the entry of the penis into the vagina, but female orgasm is actually more likely to be achieved by clitoral stimulation than by thrusting away in the manner beloved of simple-minded pornography. If you are a man and the idea that sex and penetration are not the same thing seems unusual to you, you are sadly not alone.

Perhaps the roots of this inability to give women what they want lie in childhood when, as we have seen, physical contact is largely confined to the bruising shocks of sports day, and emotional openness is seen as weakness and an excuse for bullying. Men are taught as children that there is something dirty about the genitals. Touching them, and touching other people is, in our society at least, seen as an inherently feminine thing to do. Between boys sex is either not mentioned or relegated to toilets and bike sheds where it is an all-male and jocular activity. Because girls are supposed to be pure and good, talking about sex with women is out of the question. Sexual technique is learned from soft porn and those televised bedroom scenes in which women are driven to the limits of desire by a little bit of frenzied groping. Given all this, it is hardly surprising that male insensitivity and the perfunctory nature of sex-play is cited by many women as the main reason why they find their relationships sexually unfulfilling.

A lot of the problem is rooted in the notion of foreplay, which is fundamentally flawed. This is because it sounds like something you should do before sex, a necessary prerequisite like putting on your shoes before you go for a walk. Instead of the automatic, ritualised behaviour that most men think of as foreplay – breasts, nipples, clitoris, enter, sums up many a technique – it is better to aim for sensuality, the enjoyment of every part of your lover's body. Foreplay *is* sex, then, and as such the "fore" needs to be removed, leaving simple play.

It is difficult for men to listen to such ideas because they invest their sexual prowess with so much significance. Being good at sex – being a good technician – is something that men are, and if they aren't good at it then they are somehow not real men at all. As real men should be able to give pleasure to women by penetration alone (or so the myth has it) resorting to masturbation or cunnilingus is an admission of failure. Many women seem to believe this as well, and prefer to fake an orgasm to keep their lovers content rather than threatening their egos by asking for something different. Everything conspires to allow the poor workman to go on praising his tool.

There are four things any man can start doing today to improve his sex life and make it more fulfilling. They are:

- *Talk:* ask your partner what she wants and tell her what you like.
- *Touch:* caress, hug and lie close to your partner, whether or not you are about to have sex.
- *Relax:* abandon goal-directed foreplay for sensual exploration of each other's bodies.
- *Invent:* if sex is a routine, change the way or the place or the time you make love.

For many men making these changes will take courage. They may involve overcoming emotional barriers that have been in place since early childhood. Remedies that may help at different stages of the process include:

- Chicory for the man who feels offended and rejected at the thought that his lover might not enjoy sex with him as much as he thought.
- Crab Apple for the man who feels unclean or disgusted at the thought of certain types of sexual behaviour such as cunnilingus, mutual masturbation or even simple touching.
- Gentian for the man who feels discouraged following a setback, and thinks about giving up and going back to the way things were before.
- Heather for the man who is so wrapped up with what he wants out of sex that he isn't able to listen to his partner's needs.
- Larch for the man who would like to try to be a better lover but is convinced that he will not succeed.
- Mimulus for the man who is scared of broaching the subject at all.

- Red Chestnut for the man who hesitates because he is afraid that his lover's feelings will be hurt if he tries to make changes.
- Pine for the man who feels guilty about his attitudes or behaviour yet seems trapped in this feeling and unable to take positive action.
- Rock Water for the man who is too obsessed with sheer technical perfection to remember that sex is about emotions as well as bodies.
- Wild Rose for the man who may acknowledge the need for change but is resigned to staying as he is.

Of course, the personality and reactions of any one man might be very different to any of those listed above, and some individuals may need different remedies or even none at all if there are no emotional problems. Everyone is different, in sex as in everything else. Self-discovery is one of the great rewards of a fulfilling sex life just as it is at the heart of the Bach philosophy.

CHAPTER 3

IN AND OUT
OF LOVE

FALLING IN LOVE

By the age of 16 or 17, girls will have assumed a greater importance
in the minds of most adolescent boys. Some teenagers will begin
dating, others may have been doing so already for some time, while
others still may feign indifference or be too wrapped up in some
other activity to give sex and love much thought. But the bodily
changes gone through put the question of pairing off firmly on the
agenda sooner or later, meaning that a whole new language and set
of behaviour patterns have to be learned.

Thanks to his training the average man will start off with little
idea what women want or how to go about appealing to them. He
will most likely be fully aware of his inexperience, but the macho
need to appear experienced and devil-may-care about such things
may prevent him from seeking help in the obvious ways, such as
asking women for advice or simply approaching the woman in
whom he is interested in an honest and straightforward way. Instead
emotional insecurities are usually suffered alone or with the
doubtful support of other males in his peer group. Fortunately the
Bach Flower Remedies can be helpful at such times, not only to raw
adolescents but also to older people who are having problems
making friends with potential partners.

Lack of confidence is a common problem. If the would-be lover
finds it hard to tell the object of his passion about his feelings, Larch
would be the remedy to choose. If he is overweight and feels himself
unattractive for this reason, or has some physical defect and fears
rejection because of this, then Crab Apple might help. Then there is

the person who knows whom he wants and has a fair idea how to approach her but still distrusts his judgement. He will often go around asking everyone he can think of for their opinions of this or that plan of conquest, each more cunning than the last. Meanwhile of course the object of this plotting is unaware of his interest so that there is a real risk that he will miss his chance entirely. Cerato would be his remedy.

Where an approach has been made and rejected a number of reactions are possible. Self-pity or resentment would call for Willow, hatred and jealousy would need Holly, while depression would need Gentian or Gorse depending on the severity of the emotions experienced. The young man who resigned himself to his fate and gave up trying would need Wild Rose. A pretence that the rejection did not matter, where this covered a hurt inside, would call for Agrimony. In some cases, where the ego has been bruised unexpectedly or particularly badly, Star of Bethlehem might be needed to help cope with the shock of rejection.

Fortunately not all declarations of interest in someone are unsuccessful, but the effects of success can in certain circumstances be as disruptive and potentially negative. Some people invest everything in their love affairs and can easily ignore other matters like eating, sleeping and working. This is especially true of teenagers, whose feelings are very intense anyway. This combined with awakening sexuality and the wild mood swings they can go through at this age make for a potent combination. Clematis could be used to keep the person's feet on the ground so that he would not entirely give up all his old friends, interests and studies while dreaming of love. Exams, university places and promotion at work have their own logic and a place must be left for them, however dull the necessity might seem to the ardent lover.

Of course, things are often not even as cut and dried as this. Some people find it hard to decide whether they feel attracted to someone or not, or even which of two potential partners they are more interested in. First one option seems right then, within minutes, the other seems to be the one to choose. For such people Scleranthus is the remedy to help clear away the clouds of uncertainty.

LONELINESS

Sometimes the search for a partner goes on a long time and is fruitless. Perhaps there was a relationship but it has ended prematurely. Or maybe a man has been so busy building his career and chasing material success that he is left on the shelf and finds himself still on his own long after his old friends have settled down. Whatever the cause of loneliness, it is a hard thing to bear.

Dr Bach grouped three of his flower remedies under the heading 'loneliness'. They are not the only remedies from which to choose when selecting for someone who is feeling lonely, but they are in most cases among the first to be considered. The remedies are Heather, Impatiens and Water Violet.

The main characteristics of the Heather man are that he is talkative, concerned with his own worries to the exclusion of everyone else's, and scared of being on his own. He is the man who corners you at a party and drones on about himself for hours at a time. It is for this reason that Dr Bach referred to people of this type as 'buttonholers'. The Heather man becomes emotional quite easily and will cry more readily than the majority of men – but always it is his own situation that drives him to tears, for he has little time for other people's problems. If you try to tell him about the things that worry you he will hardly even seem to hear.

The central irony of the Heather man is that his behaviour in itself is enough to bring about the outcome he fears. For his preoccupation with himself and his constant chatter are hard for other people to take and they soon start trying to avoid him. Scared of being isolated, then, the Heather man finds it hard to hold on to friends and has little chance of establishing new relationships. With the help of the Heather remedy, the hope is that this vicious cycle can be arrested. Better balanced, the Heather type turns into a good listener who is all the better at sympathising with others because of the pain in his own life. As he is better company, he finds it easier to make and keep friends so that loneliness is avoided more effectively.

Heather people are very different from the second type, Impatiens. Where the first are eager to get attention from others, the second are in most cases happy to avoid it because it slows them down. Impatiens men are generally very quick mentally, able to grasp new ideas rapidly and with little effort. They do everything as speedily as possible and feel immense waves of frustration and irritation when other people slow them down by asking for help, explanation and second thoughts.

Loneliness can come when they have so successfully cut themselves off from potential irritation that they find themselves working and living alone. A sometimes brusque manner added to tapping feet, twiddling fingers and frequent glances at watches and clocks can serve as all-too-effective people-repellents. The role of the remedy, then, is to bring a measure of patience and human sympathy to the feverish world of the Impatiens man so that he can find time for others and for his own emotional needs.

Water Violet is the third of Dr Bach's three remedies for loneliness. It is aimed at those who actually enjoy being alone, not because it allows them to do things faster, but because they really do enjoy their own company. Self-possessed and self-reliant they are not selfish so much as disinterested, preferring to go their own way rather than get entangled in the problems of others.

There is nothing at all wrong with this, of course, and many Water Violet people are happy, independent and not in need of treatment by the Bach Flower Remedies or anything else. The remedies are only called on when the Water Violet man finds, usually quite suddenly, that he has managed to lose contact with the rest of the human race. He can no longer choose to enjoy his own company because his own is the only company he has. When this happens the remedy is there to help him to unbend and admit his need for love and friendship. He will not seem so aloof, and those who have dismissed him as proud and stand-offish will come to see that he is still a good and gentle man and someone well worth getting to know.

These then are the three remedies that Dr Bach said were specifically for a form of loneliness, and we can now see that what he meant was that these were personality types who were faced with loneliness more often than most because of their natures. As the Bach Flower Remedies always aim to treat the root cause of a problem the 'loneliness' remedies would not necessarily be used where loneliness was a symptom growing out of another cause, which again would usually be found rooted in the individual's personality type. For example, someone with a very possessive nature could be lonely because the demands he makes on his loved ones have actually driven them away from him. In his case Chicory would be the type remedy to choose. On the other hand that person who accepts his loneliness with a shrug, never going out or inviting anyone to his house or making any other effort to make friends could be a Wild Rose type and so Wild Rose would be the type remedy around which to base a complete treatment.

Wild Rose can provide a good example of the use of helper or mood remedies as additions to the main type remedy. The Chicory person in the previous paragraph might feel as apathetic about life as the Wild Rose type, but in his case Wild Rose would be given in addition to Chicory since the apathy is an associated mental state brought on by loneliness rather than the cause of it. Similarly, the sense of being alone might lead someone to sink into depression, in which case Gentian, Gorse or Sweet Chestnut would also be considered as possible helper remedies, depending on the strength of the depression.

Other remedies that might help in particular cases could include:

- Willow for self-pity or resentment at the happiness of those who are enjoying relationships.
- Crab Apple for dislike of oneself.
- Larch for any loss of confidence that impedes the effort to make friends.
- Walnut for the lonely person who is kept in a rut because unwanted circumstances, habits or other influences make it hard for him to meet others.
- Honeysuckle for the person who retreats into the past.
- Clematis for his brother who daydreams of great deeds in the future instead of facing today's problems.

BREAKING UP

The early days of a relationship are full of hope and optimism. Unfortunately that optimism is often ill-placed, and as the stresses and strains of everyday living take their toll many relationships buckle and eventually break. Divorce can be particularly traumatic since not only is a couple splitting up, but households and whole families. When there are children the pain is obviously all the greater, with the children suffering as much or more than the adults. In any case the process of decay in a relationship is usually a long-drawn-out one, with many signs of trouble in the months and years leading up to the end.

One of the most avoidable of these early problems is jealousy. Judging by their behaviour many men have a real fear that their wives or girlfriends are seeing someone else, a fear which often seems out of all proportion to any actual evidence of unfaithfulness. The main remedy against these negative emotions is Holly, especially where there is anger and hatred involved, but as always other remedies could be indicated depending on the personality and individual responses of the man in question. Chicory would be used where it seems that a possessive, selfish man is using his suspicions as a means of keeping his partner under his immediate control. Mimulus would be the remedy for the straightforward fear of losing a loved one, which could be at the root of possessive behaviour. For the person who is troubled by unwanted jealous thoughts White Chestnut might be indicated, or Crab Apple if the thoughts are obsessive and need to be cleansed entirely.

Sometimes of course jealousy is well-founded. The remedies already suggested could still be useful in particular cases, as the need to think things through and behave rationally is, if anything, even greater in such circumstances. To deal with depression caused by an unfaithful lover Gentian or Gorse would be the first choice. Any loss of confidence could be helped with Larch, or Elm where a normally secure and responsible person suddenly feels unable to cope. Cherry Plum is the remedy for the fear of losing self-control, and would be indicated for those who feel that their suspicions might lead them to do an injury to their partners or to themselves.

Like jealousy, guilt can be a problem irrespective of whether anyone is really to blame or not. People can blame themselves for the things their partners have done as much as for their own actions, and self-blame like this can lead to a great deal of unhappiness.

Guilt is a necessary emotion as long as it is constructive – if you are able to learn lessons from the bad way you feel, alter your behaviour, then carry on with your life. But where guilt lasts beyond this point or where you have actually done nothing wrong and do not deserve to feel guilty, then it can be a wholly destructive emotion that prevents you from enjoying other relationships or anything else in your life. For this poisonous type of guilt Pine is the remedy to choose, whether or not you originally had anything to feel guilty about.

Other remedies that are often called on when a relationship ends include:

- Agrimony for those who seem to go on as normal but inside are suffering mental torture.
- Willow for feelings of self-pity, bitterness and resentment, either against a partner or against other couples who have been luckier in love.
- Mimulus for a fear of the future.
- Red Chestnut for those who are paralysed by concern over the effect the break-up will have on their partners or children.
- Mustard for those black depressions that can come from nowhere, when everything seems pointless.
- Holly for hatred and jealousy.
- Gorse for feelings of despair and hopelessness.
- Wild Rose to counteract any tendency to let yourself go and drift without trying to start again.
- Scleranthus where the ability to make decisions seems to have been lost, so that you find it difficult to get your life moving again.

After any break-up, but especially after a divorce involving children and the division of a home, there will be a great deal of readjusting to do. The male partner is usually the one who moves away from the family home, and after a divorce the wife almost always gets custody of the children and often the home as well. For a father, this means less contact with his children as well as the need to get used to living in a new place and the loss of all kinds of possessions and old ways of life. Walnut is the remedy to help you adjust to and live with these changes with as little pain as possible. If nostalgia for the relationship makes it hard to give sufficient attention to the things you need to sort out now, then Honeysuckle might also help.

Men who are unsure of their ability to cope with the changes caused by a break-up might be helped by Larch, or by Elm if they are normally very reliable and capable people who are suffering a temporary overload. Loneliness can also be a problem for men who find themselves living alone again after many years as a couple. Often they will be living away from family members and their old friends are either scattered far and wide or too busy with their own lives to spare time for the newly-single man. Men missing the affection they used to enjoy as the centre of a close family might need Chicory. Heather would be the remedy for men whose fear of loneliness makes them over-talkative. Their constant chatter about themselves can become a barrier to real friendship, so that the remedy gift of better emotional balance is a prerequisite to their being able to communicate in a meaningful way. For the opposite type, those quiet, self-contained people who enjoy their own company but who can find it hard to become friendly with new people, Water Violet might be the remedy to choose.

DOMESTIC VIOLENCE

There are some relationships that seem to be founded on hate and violence rather than love, and in such cases the ending of the relationship may be the most positive thing about it. In the overwhelming majority of cases the violent partner is the male – unsurprisingly, perhaps, since so many boys are taught from childhood that physical strength and dominance are the answer to life's problems. As might be expected, the men most likely to be violent in their personal relationships are those who were themselves the victims of violent fathers, or who saw their fathers beating their mothers.

Because the problems are often deep-rooted and very difficult to resolve, and because women in a violent home are at real risk of injury, it is very important to seek help at an early stage if domestic violence is becoming a problem. There are associations and women's groups set up specifically to address this problem, and help is also available from local social service agencies, doctors and community organisations. The perpetrators of violence can get help as well as the victims – often they are as trapped in the cycle of domestic cruelty as their victims are.

As far as the Bach Flower Remedies are concerned the key to helping a violent man to understand and deal with his emotional and mental problems lies once more in finding the correct remedy to address his personality defects and the transient emotional states that come with them. For the man whose jealousy or hatred, either of his wife or of the world in general, leads him to lash out in violent outbursts, Holly would be the obvious remedy to choose. Cherry Plum would also be a help where violent episodes were characterised by loss of control or where someone feared committing violent acts while in this state.

Other men might benefit from Vine, the remedy for those whose desire for dominance and assumption of authority will not stand for any resistance. People of this type have a tendency to be cruel and unnecessarily hard on others and they may resort to violence if they feel it is the simplest way of getting what they want. In yet other cases the violent acts might seem genuinely out of character. It can be worth looking then for some episode in the person's past which caused a shock that has never been resolved satisfactorily. For example, the shock of seeing your father attack your mother might stay with you, repressed deep in your psyche, yet come out in a repetition of the pattern in your own adult life. Star of Bethlehem would be a useful remedy if you feel that something of this kind might partly explain a violent man's behaviour: the remedy will deal with old, unassimilated shocks as well as it will deal with new ones.

Many people find it difficult to sympathise with a violent man, and it is of course understandable and right that most people's concern and care will be directed first at his victims. If there is to be a successful intervention using the remedies, however, it is essential to understand the person's character. Without some attempt at empathy this will be almost impossible. The thing to remember is that men are rarely in control of their violent impulses and may be as puzzled and distressed by them as their victims are.

Although it is true, as has been said, that women are the main victims of domestic violence there are still some cases where men are victimised by violent women. It might even be a more common problem than is supposed, because men will often not attract attention to bullying at home. It hardly fits in with the ideal of the manly man to admit that you are terrorised by your wife, and generations of laughter at the expense of hen-pecked husbands make most men very eager to avoid any complaints that might cast them in this role.

The classic hen-pecked husband is the Centaury man. He is a born helper and always eager to be of service – not at all like the stereotypical macho man. When he falls into the clutches of a stronger and more dominant personality his willing assistance can turn to virtual slavery. At his most unassertive he will not stand up for himself even under physical assault. The aim of the Centaury remedy for such people is not to get them to be more aggressive, but simply to restore their power to resist unfair pressure and intimidation – in other words, to restore the ability to say 'no'.

A different type of male victim is the man who tries to get on with his life as stoically as he can without reacting too much to violence at home. He shows courage in endurance but his steady approach is not always the best way of resolving the problem. In fact it may even goad his partner on to more attacks simply because she wants to provoke a response. The type remedy for such a man might well be Oak, although there would be some argument for trying Chestnut Bud as well if he seemed to be failing to learn from past experience that suffering in silence is usually not the best way to resolve such issues.

What is written here about victims and perpetrators alike might suggest that domestic violence is only ever carried out or suffered by particular types of people. Of course this is not true. Anyone may find an outlet for his personal frustrations by hitting out at a partner, just as anyone can be the partner of someone who does the hitting. As always the Dr Bach method is to treat the individual, and to that extent the remedies suggested here (and elsewhere in this and other books) are for guidance only. They do not replace direct and personal knowledge of the people being treated.

This chapter has provided an opportunity to look in more detail at the way certain remedies match up with particular mental states and personalities, and at the way type and helper remedies can be combined with each other to produce more complete solutions. As the rest of this book will show the general principles outlined here hold true for other situations that men find themselves in. And in none of these situations will the remedies find more to do than in the emotional cauldron that men call work.

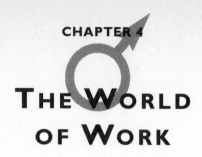

CHAPTER 4

THE WORLD
OF WORK

CHOOSING A CAREER AND GETTING A JOB

In many ways work can be a liberator. It puts money in the pocket. It provides independence and status. And almost regardless of the nature of the job and the youth of the person doing it the rest of the world recognises a worker as an adult. In return he is expected to show more self-discipline and, in the words of the Bible, to put away childish things.

Nowadays, and for the majority of people leaving school or university, starting the first full-time job is not the wrench it might appear to be from the outside. This is because most people will have amassed a fair amount of work experience already, starting with a paper round at thirteen and going on to Saturday jobs in super-markets and so on at fifteen and sixteen. This will have given them practice in the basic skills of holding down employment, such as arriving on time, taking instruction from superiors and juggling a budget from one pay-day to the next.

The crucial difference between Saturday jobs and full-time work can be summed up in a single word: seriousness. Saturday jobs are known to be temporary and there is little fall-out if things don't work. The money is typically spent on going out, computer games and clothes, and while it may be inconvenient to do without these things schoolboys do not lose their homes or go without food if they lose or leave a job. Most important of all their current jobs do not have any effect on their future prospects. In other words the likelihood of becoming a doctor or a lawyer depends on more than the fact that you spend your weekends stacking shelves or waiting on table.

This changes when full-time work starts. At first there is little danger of not eating and not having a place to live, since most people will still be living with their parents. And even if they are living alone parents are usually there to provide a refuge if things do not work out. But career prospects are affected at once, and as soon as you accept a job you are restricting your future. In other words the more labouring jobs you do the harder it will be to convince someone that you would make a good accountant, because employers nearly always look for consistency in a career and prefer people who can show that they have had a long-standing interest in the jobs they are trying to get.

The problem for many is knowing what they actually want to do with their lives. Years ago this was less of an issue since sons typically followed fathers or had their decisions made for them. For the well-born boy this might mean a career in the army, church or politics; for the lower class boy an apprenticeship to a recognised craftsman or a life spent doing physical work. Few ever got the chance to experience the angst of wondering what to be; but on the other hand freedom was limited and it was harder to be yourself. Not many people would willingly go back to such times, and nowadays the Centaury remedy is often recommended for people who are unable to stand up to the dictates of parents or teachers and because of this are led into careers that give them neither pleasure nor fulfillment.

Where doubt as to the career to follow is a problem, help is available – from schools and universities, as well as the Careers Service, Jobcentres and all kinds of other agencies. A trip to the local library can also provide endless books on the different careers that you might want to follow, from circus juggler to small businessman to electrical engineer. And most people will find that a little thought and research into who they are will also suggest possible careers.

First of all, the school-leaver looking for the right career could ask himself what things he likes and dislikes doing. If he hates crowds and noise and dislikes being the centre of attention he is probably not suited to a career teaching secondary schoolchildren but might enjoy a research job or work in an office. If he has a hobby or is fascinated by a subject, is there any way to find a job that would be an extension of it? Even if his main interest seems entirely passive, such as watching historical dramas on TV or listening to CD's, there might still be a job to be had at a theatrical costumiers, a television production company, a music shop or a concert hall. Then there is the question of how he responds to pressure, to stress, to the idea of conflict at work and to responsibility. There is little point in his chasing after a high-pressure sales job if it is going to leave him upset and exhausted at the end of every day. It is usually a mistake to force oneself to fit in with organisations and ways of working that are entirely foreign to one's personality. If you don't get something more than money out of your time at work you will end up doing a bad job and hating a third of your life.

People who have already defined their type remedy under the Bach system are well on their way to knowing the answers to some of these questions. Other conundrums are more mundane and depend on personal circumstances more than personality: how long will it be possible to wait for the right job to come along before being forced by financial pressures to take a wrong one, for instance? And is it practical to consider the perfect job if it means moving to another area? Ideally questions of this kind will not have as much weight as the more long-term ones, but they may still be important.

Even after all this there are some people who seem to go from school to a succession of jobs with little sense of direction or purpose. Sometimes sheer apathy is the cause, a feeling of resignation and fatality that causes the person to drift through life shrugging his shoulders and saying that this is just the way things are and that there is nothing he can do (or rather, be bothered to do) to change them. Wild Rose is the remedy to wake such people up a little so that they can take more interest in life and in themselves.

The Wild Rose man will be dulled to his condition and so suffers correspondingly less from it. The person in a Wild Oat state, however, is not at all resigned. He feels greatly dissatisfied with what he is doing and the direction his life is taking. He may be someone who has always seemed talented and for whom great things were forecast. Yet as he steps out into life he loses his way. He knows he wants to do something worthwhile and leave the world changed and better for his having been there. But he cannot see which way he should go and so, like the Wild Rose, he drifts. He goes from job to job, always trying different things and never finding his true path. For him, the Wild Oat remedy is the one to lift the fog of indecision so that he can see the way ahead clearly and start to fulfill his tremendous potential.

There are similarities between the Wild Oat person and the next type of career-seeker, the one in the Chestnut Bud state, since both of them typically do a whole string of different jobs. But where the Wild Oat chops and changes career the Chestnut Bud seems unable to learn from his past errors. He will quit his first job in disgust, vowing never to work in an office again, and two weeks later will apply for another job working in an almost identical office. The remedy in this case is to help him stop the cycle of repetition and disappointment. He also needs encouragement to look within himself and start looking for the things he does want to do.

Of course, nothing – and certainly not the Bach Flower Remedies – can make someone a success in a particular career if he lacks the basic skills needed to do the job. So as well as analysing who he is and what he wants to do, the career-hunter needs to look at his strengths and weaknesses when it comes to actually doing a job – and applying for it.

In many cases you should review your skills before you start applying for jobs. In other words there are a large number of careers where there is no point perfecting interview techniques if the knowledge necessary to do the job is lacking. Nine times out of ten the answer to a shortage of skills lies in some kind of training, and it doesn't have to be formal or lead to a paper qualification. Many necessary skills from touch typing to book-keeping to car maintenance can be learnt with the help of the local library and a certain amount of application. Local adult education centres are also good places to learn all kinds of extra skills that will look good on a CV. The fees are usually low and there are often reductions for the unemployed and people on low income. Most centres will also provide free tuition in basic numeracy and literacy for those who need it.

Where formal qualifications are necessary for a career, the first step is to find out what those qualifications are. Outside the realms of medicine and the law, which tend to stick to quite rigid examination structures, there are usually many ways to get started. Indeed in many professions it doesn't much matter what someone has studied as long as he has studied something successfully and to the required level. The computer industry, for example, is full of people with degrees in art, 'A' levels in Latin and GCSE economics. Some of the top designers of computer games have no formal computing qualifications at all.

People who have contacts in the sector in which they want to work should use them. The career-seeker can ask his contacts how they got started and what they did to get their first chance and then try the same himself. Those who don't know anyone can make their own contacts. One trick is to phone up the switchboard of a company operating in the selected industry and ask for the name of the person who does the job you want. It's probably best not to speak to him at this stage as he is almost certainly busy and may not welcome an interruption. Instead, a polite and enthusiastic letter can be written saying how interested you are in what he and his company do and that you are looking to make that area your career. If you don't think your letter-writing is up to it, get a how-to book from the library. Most people will respond and at the very least will provide a few tips on what the next step should be – and there is always the chance that the letter itself will lead to an interview.

Those who have no experience in the thing they want to do and cannot find any way of gaining experience without getting the job first have no alternative but to rely entirely on their job-searching skills. This is not the place for an in-depth description of the various strategies that can be tried to make job-hunting more successful. The appendix at the back of this book lists a couple of books that do that, and there are lots more in any local library. Nevertheless it might be useful to give a brief summary of the subject, which can be broken down into three main areas, namely:

- Spotting the right vacancy.
- Getting an interview.
- Succeeding at the interview.

We have already seen some of the ways to spot the right vacancy, the most important of which was defining what the right vacancy really is. As you probably remember this involved a little self-analysis in order to find out who you are and what you really want to do. The jobs themselves might be found in newspaper and magazine advertisements, especially sections of the press specialising in the selected area, or via personal referral from friends or relatives or contacts who are already in that line of work, or posted up in Jobcentres and Careers Centres. In addition it's usually worth doing the rounds of all the areas within travelling distance, as many agencies concentrate on local vacancies only. A job in the next town or county will be listed in Jobcentres there but might not be posted up in your local office.

Getting a potential employer to offer an interview is the next hurdle. Even quite ordinary vacancies can easily attract 30 or 40 applicants these days, and it is reckoned that most CV's and application forms sent in are looked at for only 30 seconds before a decision is made as to whether to see that person for an interview or not. If there are only 30 seconds available in which to impress it is essential to make the most of them.

First of all, CV's should be kept short and to the point, and the strongest selling point should be right at the top where it is more likely to be seen. What that selling point is will depend on whether you have done the job before and what qualifications you have, and one or other of these will normally feature prominently. But other items might belong there instead. For example, a CV would not normally contain a list of hobbies at the top of page one. But someone looking for a hardware support technician will be more interested in the fact that you have just finished building your own PC than he will be in your GCSE in chemistry or your Saturday job in the fish market. You need to play on your strengths, and find the things in your past or present that will make employers think of you as a serious candidate.

Some people pay to have professional CVs put together for them and printed out on glossy paper. This may be effective for people who are going consistently for the same type of job so that they always want to stress the same qualities and gloss over the same drawbacks. But for those of us who are applying for a range of positions it is not such a good idea. Every printed CV sent off will look exactly the same no matter what employer it is sent to, so that the chance to make an individual impact and tailor the contents to an individual employer's needs is lost. It's probably better to make up your own CV afresh each time, and to aim it specifically at the job you are currently applying for. Obviously you will always check all the spelling in your CV and ensure that it is typed or printed on clean paper. If you use a typewriter or a computer with a dot matrix printer make sure you have a new ribbon in it: using a worn-out, pale ribbon may save you a few pounds but will also ensure that half the people who get your CV will put it straight on the reject pile.

Sometimes advertisements ask you to complete an application form instead of sending a CV, and in this case you are of course less free to influence what the employer will and will not read and in what order. However, you should resist the temptation to ignore the application form and send your CV in anyway. There is usually a good reason why application forms are asked for instead of CVs, and you will almost certainly exclude yourself from consideration if you annoy the person receiving applications or seem incapable of following the simplest instruction.

You need to take some time to fill out application forms, just as you would take time to put together your CV. For a start it's a good idea to read every question and instruction on the form before you fill it out. You will not impress anyone if you have written your postcode in with the rest of your address and then crossed it out when you notice the special box provided for postcodes. Nor will employers be impressed by handwriting in green biro when it specifically says at the top of the form that you should write in block capitals and use black ink. They will also react badly to people who cannot spell the name of the company they are applying to.

Almost every application form has a place where you can, if you want, provide additional information in support of your application. Many people do not fill this in, perhaps thinking that they have supplied enough information already. This is a mistake. An employer who is undecided will often turn to this section in order to make his mind up. So if you play football every Sunday or sit for hours by yourself reading, take the chance to impress potential employers with your ability to work well in a team or your capacity for concentration.

Even if you ignore this advice and don't provide additional information, at least provide the information asked for. If you leave parts of the form blank and don't provide appropriate responses to questions you will arouse the suspicions of employers who may think you are hiding something.

Once you have identified what you want to do and supplied an application form that has got you onto a short-list you will be called in for an interview. Between the day you receive the invitation to the day of the interview itself you have a chance to improve your chances by finding out a few basic facts about the company and what it does. Unless you are applying for a senior post that will involve you in determining the future direction of the company you won't be expected to have any in-depth knowledge. But you will stand out from the crowd if you are able to talk intelligently about the company's area of interest and can pitch your answers at the interview to the type of company you are talking to. If you can't find out something that too can be useful. For example, if you know the company you are looking to join has a reputation for being very traditional yet the post being offered is in a high-tech area you can demonstrate your intelligence and interest in the company by asking the obvious question.

Much of the information you need will come from the advertisement that you originally replied to. More will be found in material that the company sends you along with the letter offering you an interview. You can also ask your local library if they hold information on local businesses. If you know someone who works for the company already then you have an especially privileged source of information and you should make the most of it.

Of course, there is no point researching the company if you then spoil everything by turning up for the interview late or badly dressed.

Aim to arrive 15 minutes before the set time, and err on the side of caution. If you will be travelling to an area that you don't know well you should try to do a dry run to check the route, journey times, where you can park and so on. If you haven't got the time for a dry run then you should aim to arrive an hour early and make sure you have an accurate map of where you have to go. That way you have time to get lost a couple of times without unnecessary panic.

As for clothes, a suit, shirt and tie are pretty much expected for office jobs, and for manual jobs a shirt and tie will usually help to make a good first impression. Of course, you might have information that makes you think this will be inappropriate, and some sectors such as advertising, fashion and design are known to be less formal than others. Even in these cases you should aim to be clean and presentable.

Once the interview has actually started there are a number of standard questions that you can expect to be asked, and in each case there is a right and a wrong way to respond to them. For example:

- 'Did you have any trouble finding us?'
  The correct answer is always 'no', because you are well-organised and allowed enough time to get there early.
- 'Do you know anything about this company?'
  Yes you do, because you've done some research. Say what you know and mention anything that particularly interests you about the company's philosophy or its current activities.
- 'Why do you want this job?'
  You might mention that you want to work for a progressive/traditional company, or that you are particularly committed to the company's policy on the environment/community schemes/basic research or whatever. This is also a chance to mention your ambitions to learn more and improve yourself. Whatever you answer, don't just say you want the money because that makes people think you are not interested in making a commitment to the company. They might also suspect that you will leave as soon as you are offered a little more to work somewhere else.
- 'What special qualities can you bring to this job?'

You will have identified your strong and your weak points, and now is the time to dwell on the former. Make sure that you slant everything you say to the requirements of the job itself.

- 'I see from your application form that (etc.)... Won't this be a disadvantage in this job?'

  Like you the interviewer will have gone through your CV highlighting your weak points. You need to be prepared to give a positive slant to them. For example, if you have no previous experience of the job you are trying to get you could emphasise your willingness to learn and the fact that you would listen to the company's way of doing things rather than following inappropriate procedures that you learnt somewhere else.

The one thing all these answers have in common is that they are all attempting to give the interviewer the kind of answer he or she wants. Having thought about the job you are trying for and knowing a bit about the company you are in a better position than most to come up with sensible responses.

At some stage of the interview, usually at the end, you will be asked if there are any questions that you want to ask yourself. This is the verbal equivalent of the 'any further information' section on an application form, and again the advice is to take advantage of the opportunity to make a good impression. Not asking anything or saying rather lamely that everything has already been covered makes it look as if you just want to get out of the door as soon as possible. Good questions you could ask include what potential there is for promotion and/or training, what the future prospects of the company are in terms of new products or growth, and how the job you are applying for fits in with others in the company structure. Don't overdo things, however, because the chances are the person interviewing you has other people to see and has only allowed a few minutes for your questions. It's all right to ask about money and holidays if they haven't been covered already, but probably best not to make this your only question as it makes it look as if you are only interested in what you can get out of the company.

Even well-prepared interviewees can still suffer from the stresses and strains of the process. These can lead to distracting behaviour during the interview itself, such as fidgeting around or being unable to make eye contact with the person asking the questions. They can even cause you to forget the answers you have prepared and gloss over your best points just so that you can get out of the room a bit faster. The Bach Flower Remedies can come in very useful for dealing with such problems so that you are always in control and able to make a good impression. For example:

- Fear of the interview or shyness would require Mimulus.
- Agrimony would be given for mental turbulence repressed behind a cheerful exterior.
- Larch is for lack of confidence.
- Elm would be useful if you are normally capable and sure of yourself but feel overwhelmed because so much rides on your getting a particular job.
- If you are very enthusiastic and trying too hard and this leads to your becoming tense and anxious, Vervain would be the remedy to select.
- Rescue Remedy would be a useful standby for last minute nerves or anxiety.

After the interview you may get the job or you may not. If you don't it is important not to be too downhearted. Only one person can be chosen out of all those who are interviewed and next time you might be the lucky one. Gentian is the remedy to overcome any discouragement you feel that might hamper your search in the future. If you have failed several times at interview stage it's worth taking a fresh look at your interview technique to see if you are doing something you shouldn't be doing, or not doing something you should. Chestnut Bud is the remedy to help you learn from repeated mistakes, so this might come in useful at such times.

STRESS AND OVERWORK

Not so long ago people thought that as more and more work was done by machines so people would need to do less. It was even suggested that the main problem for late 20th century man would be finding ways to fill up his increasing leisure time. The reality has proved rather different, however. The trend in Britain and many other Western countries is for employees and employers alike to work longer hours than ever before.

Opinion is divided as to why this should be so. Some blame recession and job insecurity, which cause those lucky enough to have jobs to work harder than anyone else so as to make sure they are not top of the next redundancy list. Another suggestion is that by enabling us to produce more in a shorter space of time automation has made more demands on the human side of the production process, forcing people to run harder to keep up. Yet others blame the need to compete in a global market against the cut-rate wage costs in other countries, or see longer hours as evidence that there is a shortage of appropriate skills, so that the few who have the ability to do a particular job end up doing the work of two or three people.

Whatever the social cause of the problem there is no doubt about the effect on individual workers. Stress, stress-related illnesses and overwork are more common now than at any time in human history. They have turned out to be the price paid for industrial progress, economic success and material wealth.

That this should be so is in some ways ironic, because far from being a recent phenomenon, stress is actually an age-old response by the body to danger. Its roots are in the so-called fight or flight response which gears the body up to taking quick, decisive action when it needs to deal with some threat. Adrenalin is released to pump more blood to the muscles and brain, while at the same time less blood flows to the skin so that there will be less bleeding if the body is wounded. Eyes and ears are fine-tuned to pick up more information, and the whole body assumes a state of tension, ready to act. These changes are of course aimed at taking care of a physical threat, and if someone attacks you in the street they are appropriate as you will be able to defend yourself (or run away) more effectively. And of course in taking a physical action – fighting or running – you are working off the adrenalin and its effects so that you return afterwards to your normal physical state.

Stress can be caused by almost anything. Running for a bus, hearing a car backfire and receiving a large credit card bill all cause stress in their own way. Family life too is no haven, as personality clashes and petty disagreements have their own effects on your stress levels. And the problems caused by excessive levels of stress vary as widely as the causes. They can include anxiety, asthma, depression, indigestion, heartburn, insomnia, high blood pressure and tension. In addition a wide range of complaints are made worse or triggered by stress even though they have other recognised physical causes as well. The list here ranges from relatively minor problems such as colds and 'flu, skin complaints and headaches, all the way to potentially life-threatening diseases such as heart failure, ulcers and cancer. Indeed, Dr Vernon Coleman has written (in *Stress and Relaxation*) that up to 95 per cent of illnesses 'can be blamed at least partly (and in some cases wholly) on stress'.

There are two main reasons why modern man is particularly at risk from stress. On the one hand the body's way of dealing with stress-producing stimuli is no longer appropriate. Watching a thriller on TV will cause many of the same physical responses as the same situation in real life. Adrenalin will flow when your boss tells you to get an urgent order out on time, or when you hear rumours of redundancy. But you can't fight the television, or run away from your boss, or square up to an imaginary redundancy notice. So instead of working off the effects of the stimuli the body has to learn to live with them. The result is increased physical wear and tear and less resistance to disease.

The second problem peculiar to our age is the sheer amount of stimulus all around us. Advertising, entertainment, fashion, travel all owe their impact (and a great deal of their appeal) to the fact that they cause stress, making us feel more alive and alert. This would be fine if such stresses were few and far between, but today they come at us in relentless waves. There is no escape, so that it is all too easy for the fight-or-flight state to seem normal. Once again the result is physical and mental exhaustion, that constant feeling of edginess and hurry that so many of us live with every day.

But most men would agree that the stresses associated with entertainment and advertising are relatively minor compared with the stress of work. And there seems little doubt that work is probably the single main cause of preventable stress among men of working age. According to *The Family Friendly Workplace*, a report published by the recruitment organisation Austin Knight in October 1995, 81 per cent of British men questioned worked 40 hours or more per week and more than a third worked more than 50 hours. (56 per cent of working women work 40 hours a week, 13 per cent work 50 hours.) Among senior managers conditions were even worse, and 45 per cent said they worked 50 hours or more. These figures are all the more worrying because occupations are on the whole more sedentary than they used to be, so that there is less opportunity to work off the physical effects of stress. Couple this with our expectations that we will earn and consume more and more each year and you have a recipe for disaster. It is hardly surprising that millions of working days are lost every year due to stress-related illnesses brought on by overwork and the unbearable pressure to succeed.

There are two ways that the Bach Flower Remedies can help to deal with stress and the effects of overwork. The first and simplest is to use them to deal with acute problems that demand quick solutions. The obvious first choice in many such cases would be Rescue Remedy, since this contains the five individual remedies that will help deal with many of the immediate stress-related problems encountered at work: Star of Bethlehem for shock; Rock Rose for terror; Impatiens for intense irritation, agitation and excitability; Clematis for faintness; and Cherry Plum for loss of control and hysteria. Rescue Remedy can be carried around in the pocket and four drops sipped from a glass of water will quickly relieve these symptoms whenever a crisis at work causes them.

Where the individual remedies are available, there is room to be more specific in choosing a treatment so as to aim a remedy or combination of remedies at the particular emotional problem being dealt with. Overwork leading to tiredness could be helped using Olive, for example, while people who are being held back for some reason and so feel frustrated and irritated might benefit from Impatiens.

This leads on to the second way that the remedies can help. Instead of crisis management – taking Impatiens when you feel impatient or Olive when you feel tired – it is possible (and advisable) to go deeper into the problem. Is Impatiens your type remedy, in that impatience and doing things quickly is one of your characteristics? Or is the impatience you feel a symptom of some more fundamental emotional state – resentment, for example, or guilt? In the first case Willow would be the remedy to choose, while for guilt you would be more likely to benefit from Pine. Similarly, is your tiredness a chronic problem caused by your inability to say no when your boss asks you to do yet one more extra job (Chicory), or do you feel tired because your enthusiasm has led you to take on too much (Vervain)? Different remedies would be required in all these cases to deal with the different underlying causes. And it is only by dealing with these underlying causes – and with the work practices that commonly go with them – that a satisfactory answer to stress and overwork can be found.

When considering long-term solutions to stress management problems the first thing you need to do is understand the sort of person you are. People suffering from stress should start by taking a good hard look at the way they respond to stress and at the kind of events that lead to their becoming stressed in the first place. These are the sort of questions that might be asked in order to help this process:

- How good am I at switching off at the end of the working day?
- Are there particular occasions at work – such as meetings, deadlines or times of the month – that cause me particular stress?
- Is work interfering with my family and/or social life?
- Do I have trouble sleeping at night?
- Am I always pushed for time?
- Am I tired when I wake up in the morning?
- How many meals do I miss in a week because I am too busy to eat?
- Do I tend to take on more work even when I know I will not be able to complete it on time?
- Do I dread the thought of going back to work on Monday morning?

- Am I working to live or living to work?
- How good am I at saying 'no'?
- Are there particular people at work who have a negative effect on me? If there are, what is it about these people that I find stressful?

It is also a good idea to keep a diary of the times and occasions when you feel particularly under pressure. Over days and weeks this will build into a comprehensive picture of the kinds of situations that you find particularly stressful. As well as giving you clues as to the kinds of things you should perhaps try to avoid, you can also use this as a springboard to gain a deeper understanding of who you are – in Bach Flower Remedy terms, more information about your type. Remember that if you find a particular situation stressful it may not be because there is something inherently stressful about all situations of that type. It is more likely to be the combination of three elements – the situation itself, your personality, and the way you handle it – that have made the experience stressful. To reduce the likelihood of the stress recurring you have to understand and allow for all three elements.

Of course there is no short-cut to choosing the right remedy – you can't add up the number of 'yes' answers and arrive at an infallible prescription. But what techniques like these can do is help you to focus on your own individual personality and the way it leads you to react to potentially stressful situations at work. In this way you can pick the right remedy or group of remedies to help you. And as well as helping you choose a remedy the answers you give should help to suggest ways that you can better organise your working day so that you can discharge your responsibilities without affecting your health.

For example, someone who finds it hard to switch off and suffers from endless mental arguments might benefit from White Chestnut. This is the remedy for those people who react to stress by re-running things in their minds over and over again. A similar problem is experienced by people of the Agrimony type. Agrimony men attempt to hide their problems behind a smile, and are often so good at doing this that their work-mates can be quite shocked when they find out that things are not going as well as it seemed. Like people in the White Chestnut state, Agrimony men suffer greatly from sleeplessness since the thoughts that they repress during the day return with redoubled force late at night. In order to gain a respite they sometimes turn to drink and drugs to help drown out their worries. If this sounds like you, the Agrimony remedy can help you to face up to your worries instead of always trying to run away from them.

In either of these cases, knowing that you are a worrier can help you define a strategy to avoid and lessen the stress your worries cause you. You might decide to make a deliberate effort to share your worries with other people. You might also try setting aside a particular time every day when you will do nothing but worry – twenty minutes is usually enough – so that the rest of your time can be spent enjoying life. Whenever a worrying thought occurs you can jot it down and forget about it until your worry time starts. And by planning when and how you will worry you should find it easier to get constructive results from your worrying rather than endlessly circling around the same old tracks.

Other examples of people who are particularly prone to stress include Elm and Oak men, who can find that simply because they are good at coping with responsibility they are inclined to take on too much. Under stress, Elm people sometimes feel overwhelmed by their commitments and so begin to doubt their abilities. Oak men are slightly different in that they will carry on regardless, so that when they do break down the situation is all the worse. If you fit into either of these categories the respective remedies will not only help to restore your flagging strength and confidence, but will also help you to take a more balanced view of yourself so that you can see the dangers of assuming responsibility where you do not need to. If nothing else, you should learn how to rank the jobs you have to do in order of priority so that you do not waste time working on relatively unimportant assignments while very important or urgent tasks are left undone.

Vervain men also need to prioritise their work, since their natural enthusiasm can lead them to run headlong at tasks. They also tend to worry things to death, and once they have taken on a job they can be very reluctant to let it go again. Consequently the weight of work they are committed to just goes on increasing, and if nothing is done about it they can end up collapsing under the load. The remedy again restores a sense of balance so that more sensible decisions can be made and responsibilities delegated to others instead of being heaped on one desk.

Other remedies that might help in specific cases of work-related stress are Pine, Centaury and Rock Water. Pine is for those men who are never content with what they have achieved and who tend to take the blame for things going wrong, even when it is not their fault. Men who find it hard to say 'no' could in many cases benefit from Centaury, which is the remedy for those people who are naturally eager to help others but who find this leaves them open to exploitation by others who take advantage of their good natures. Centaury people need to learn how to be more assertive and also how to make sure their existing work schedules are taken into account before they agree to do more. This alone will spare them a great deal of unnecessary overwork and stress. Rock Water, on the other hand, is the remedy for those men who set themselves impossible standards and so put themselves under stress when they fail to meet them. Here again, the choice of this remedy indicates a need to look at related work practices so that things can go more smoothly in future. In this case the person would probably benefit from being rather kinder to himself and not binding himself to unreasonably tough deadlines. A well-earned holiday or some other planned treat is a good way to avoid stress, and once the remedy has softened the harsh attitude of the Rock Water person he will hopefully be in a position to permit himself the occasional fall from grace.

To sum up, the Bach Flower Remedies can be used in any case where overwork and stress are making working life a strain on health. The exact remedies to choose will depend as usual on the personality of the individual being treated and the way he responds to the demands placed on him. And in all cases successful stress management involves looking at the elements in your character that lead you into stressful situations. Often the long-term solution is largely a question of setting realistic goals and of learning how to delegate and prioritise tasks more effectively – in other words, it's a question of learning good time management skills. This can entail taking a hard look at the way you interact with those around you so that you can take more effective control of your own time and your own life. The aim in all cases is to bring work and the rest of your life back into balance so that both can be enjoyed in good health and happiness.

REDUNDANCY AND UNEMPLOYMENT

In the Western world an occupation is more than a means to an end, but an end in itself: when you say what you do other people decide what you are. The loss of a job is then a major trauma in the lives of most men. People who have built their personalities around their jobs may, in extreme cases, feel that they have been stripped of their identities. This man is a baker, they say, that man a butcher, while I am not doing anything.

Sometimes redundancy can strike out of the blue. This is often the case where the business is put into receivership, since the tendency among directors will be to keep the scale of the problem secret from staff and creditors in the hope that some last-minute miracle might happen. Star of Bethlehem is the remedy for all shock, including the shock of being made redundant. Rescue Remedy is also an obvious choice, and the Rock Rose in the composite is needed to control the terror – the word is not out of place – that many feel at the completely unexpected news that they will be losing their livelihoods and their security, perhaps after many years working at the same company.

Star of Bethlehem is also of use when redundancies are expected, since people will always hope that they will be spared even when colleagues have to go. They deny to themselves that they are at risk and so when the news comes it is just as shocking. Other remedies can be needed in this situation as well. In the days leading up to the actual announcements many will be in a White Chestnut state, unable to concentrate on anything because of the worries revolving without pause in their heads. Others will hide their worries under a joke and a smile, but they will not be any easier in their minds when they pause for thought, and Agrimony is the remedy for them. When a man actually receive the news that he is one of the ones to go his confidence can take a huge knock, and Larch is the remedy to restore his belief in himself and help him see that it is not his fault that things have gone wrong. It is the function within the company that is not wanted rather than the individual or his skills. Pine might be needed for those who start blaming themselves for what has happened. For resentment of those who have been lucky enough to keep their jobs Willow would be the remedy to consider.

It's important when redundancy strikes not to give way to resentment or any other negative emotions. There are several reasons for this. First, colleagues will not be feeling very happy about things whether or not they have kept their jobs, and many of them will be wondering if they are going to be next. The chances are they will be feeling just as guilty and upset as you do. There is no need to make their lives worse. On a more self-interested note there might be a possibility of the firm taking you on again if business improves or of your getting the occasional freelance assignment. You won't be considered for either if you don't adopt a positive frame of mind now. Finally, you have a great many things to do, such as claiming benefits and sorting your finances out, and you really can't afford to waste time feeling sorry for yourself.

Whether you get a large redundancy payment or not, you need to decide early on what you are going to do with the rest of your life. On the one hand, you don't want to act as if you're on holiday and spend half your money before you have worked out if you can afford to or not. On the other hand, you don't want to panic and take the first unsuitable, underpaid job you can get your hands on. Instead you need to plan. Among other things, ask yourself:

- Do I want or need to work at all?
  Starting to look for a new job can be a kind of unthinking reflex. Maybe you would be happier retiring early, or perhaps you could get by with a part-time job that would leave you time to study for another career or fulfil an ambition that work never left time for. Take some time to consider the options before you do anything.

- How much can I afford to spend?

  If you are living off a redundancy payment make plans now to deal with the day the money runs out. Get rid of your credit cards. Contact the building society, the bank and the electricity and gas companies and tell them you are out of work before you get into trouble. If you do all this early on you will feel more in control and able to get on with your life without worrying too much about money.

- What really interests me?

  Most people do jobs that don't have much to do with the things they like doing. What are the things you would do if you could, and is it possible that this is your chance to really have a go at making your dreams come true? If it is, losing your last job could be the best thing that ever happened to you.

- What are the things that are important to me?

  This is an encouragement to look at your next job and your future career in the context of everything else. If you take a high-pressure job that means travelling around far away from home, can you accept not seeing your children grow up? If you love the countryside, is it worth moving to the city to find work?

If you decide that you do want another job and have made up your mind what your priorities are and what kind of work you want to do, then you are ready to begin job hunting. Unfortunately this can be especially difficult for the newly-redundant man. He might not have been on the job market for some time and his job-search skills might be rather rusty. If the industry that he used to work in is part of a declining sector he may also find that his skills are not as highly-valued as he hoped. In this case he should certainly consider training and further education to brush up skills. This does not necessarily mean gaining formal qualifications, since often the flexibility demonstrated by the fact that you are attending some kind of career-related course will be enough to persuade an employer to give you a chance.

There is help available if you ask for it. In Britain, for example, government agencies operate a variety of schemes designed to help people find new work and new careers. Job Review Workshops help unemployed people who have been following professional and administrative careers to identify and find out about other possible career paths. There are restart schemes, job clubs, work trials and various forms of training available as well. Details of these and other schemes are available from Jobcentres. Given the fact that many of the schemes change on an almost monthly basis, with new ones being introduced all the time, it is worth asking even if you do not think that there is a scheme for people in your particular situation. Numerous self-help groups have been started too, for everyone from ex-miners to redundant middle-aged executives.

Age can also be a problem for the older job-hunter. Many firms discriminate against older applicants on the grounds that they are not as quick to learn new skills or because they think they will not be ambitious or flexible enough. The important thing is to challenge these assumptions head on and put your own view of things across right from the outset. Tell employers how you went from earning your previous salary to being redundant and how easily you coped. Stress any career changes you made earlier on and your ability to bring your wealth of experience to new challenges and how willing you are to embrace new concepts and ways of working. Talk about the range of proven basic skills you have and how you would go about adapting them to the new job. If you still don't get on the short-list it's the company which is stuck in a rut and incapable of learning, not you.

Unfortunately not everyone who wants or needs to work will be able to find work as quickly as he would like. You can help avoid the problems of prolonged unemployment if you take a few simple preventative measures. These include:

- Taking exercise.
  You will feel better about yourself – and look better too – if you take exercise regularly. (See chapter 7.)
- Taking your time.
  Accept the fact that it might take several months or even years to get the right job. Plan for an extended campaign and prepare yourself mentally to lose the odd battle along the way.

- Being kind to yourself.
  There are good sides to being out of work. You can have a lie-in when you want, you can get to know your kids, you can sit in the garden and read a novel. Don't feel guilty about these things, but enjoy them and plan them into your job-hunting schedule.
- Knowing your worth.
  Try writing down a list of all the things you are good at and all the reasons there are to think that you are a wonderful person. Practise saying them to yourself at odd moments during the day. At first it might seem a strange thing to do, but in fact all you are doing is giving yourself a boost in the same way executives do when they admire their company cars before they drive to work. The only difference is that your sense of worth comes from within you while theirs relies on an expensive prop.

All of these steps apply just as much to people who have never had a job as they do to people who have left a job or have been made redundant. In the same way the Bach Flower Remedies that apply would be of help to any of these people. For example:

- It is all too easy to become discouraged when things do not go as well as you hoped, or when a promising interview turns into another rejection letter. Gentian is the remedy to cope with such setbacks.
- Gorse would be used to cope with feeling hopeless and doubting that you will ever find the job you want.
- The emotional and mental fatigue that makes you feel too weak to get yourself going is treated with Hornbeam.
- If you get so preoccupied with your own problems that you start pouring out your troubles to all and sundry even when it is inappropriate to do so, then Heather is the remedy to help put your troubles into perspective.
- Feelings of hatred against the world for rejecting you would be eased by Holly.
- Resentment and self-pity call for Willow.

- People who feel overwhelmed by the need to provide for their family would need Elm.
- Fear that something terrible will happen to loved ones because you are out of work is a sign that Red Chestnut is needed.
- A straightforward fear of the future is a case for Mimulus.

With the help of the remedies, the support of friends and family, and the assistance of the many agencies set up to help people find work, you will succeed. It may take time, but that is something you have plenty of at the moment. Before you move on enjoy this unexpected chance to look again at who you are and where you are going.

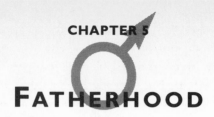

CHAPTER 5

FATHERHOOD

PREPARING FOR FATHERHOOD

Everyone knows that women have a maternal instinct, a dark and unreasoning desire to have children that will not stand for being frustrated, while men prefer not to get too involved with their children and are largely unconcerned if they do not have any.

The whole of the last paragraph is of course rubbish, but not so long ago it would have been accepted as more or less common sense. In the 1960s the idea of a father changing nappies or bathing children, let alone being present at the birth of his child, was little short of revolutionary. Yet now most fathers and would-be fathers would acknowledge that all the above are perfectly normal. Things have changed to such a degree that the father who does not want to be present at the birth of his children is considered today to be something of an oddity. The father who refuses to change a dirty nappy is simply an anachronism.

The extremes of then and now conceal the wide range of emotions that real people feel. Just as there are countless men for whom the birth of a child represents the crowning moment of their lives, so there are others who do not want children or, if they do, want to be involved in the messy end of rearing them as little as possible. There is suggestive evidence that some men suffer emotional problems if they attend the birth of their children. These can range from simple squeamishness and a loss of sexual interest in your partner to guilt at the pain she has gone through. Some men may even resent the baby for the pain she has caused her mother. For all of these emotional problems the Bach Flower Remedies may help – the first remedies to consider for physical squeamishness would probably be Crab Apple, for example, while Pine is the remedy for guilt and Willow for resentment. But prevention is better than cure, and no pressure should be put on a reluctant man to attend the birth if he is really upset at the prospect.

For most men, however, attending the birth of their children is one of the great experiences in life, and is not one to be passed up lightly. Speaking from personal experience I am sure that the birth of our two children has brought us more fulfilment and satisfaction than anything else we have gone through. Each time our relationship with each other and with the new baby was all the stronger for being shared.

In any case, the father-to-be will almost certainly face problems which he is not that well-equipped to resolve. Whereas growing girls are encouraged to show an interest in babies and the care of younger children, boys are encouraged – by other boys usually, and the ethos of the gang – not to show any interest at all. Consequently the news that he is going to be a father finds the average man singularly ill-equipped even to imagine the changes that are going to come in his life, let alone plan to deal with them. And all kinds of unexpected resentments and fears can lie below the surface, threatening to spoil the party unless they are dealt with.

When a man first learns he is to be a father there is an inevitable emotional charge to deal with. In no particular order, and depending on who he is and what the situation is, he may feel excitement, apprehension, fear, anger (perhaps he did not want a child or feels he is being deliberately trapped into a relationship), euphoria, worry, or a great swell of love for his partner and the world in general. Once things have settled down the commonest emotions left are probably anticipation and anxiety.

Of these two anticipation is usually a problem only if you are missing out on the present because you are constantly planning for the future. After all, there's little point spending nine months deciding whether little Janey or Johnny should go to Oxford or Cambridge if it stops you from helping your partner with the practicalities of nest-building. Clematis is the remedy to counteract any tendency to sacrifice the present to thoughts of tomorrow.

Anxiety is usually more of a problem. Sometimes it is centred on your partner or on the baby. Will they both get through the birth all right? How will your partner cope with being a mother? Will the baby be healthy? These are Red Chestnut fears, since they are based on an over-concern for the welfare of the people you love. The word 'over-concern' might seem strange since if you care for them how could you care too much? But the problem is that fear is a paralysing and contagious condition. Exaggerated concern may make the whole pregnancy a nightmare for you and your partner, so the remedy is used to stop this from happening.

Other fears are of specific, named possibilities. You may be afraid of the responsibility of looking after a child, or scared that you will lose (or be unable to find) the job you need in order to provide for them. Mimulus is the remedy for these known fears. It will help you face and deal with anxieties like these rather than giving in to them. So if you are anxious about money, you will be better able to analyse the fear and get help, and may be more able to look for a better-paid job. And if it is responsibility that scares you, this is a good time to learn about being a father and prepare yourself.

A third kind of fear is the vague sense of dread and impending disaster that does not have a definite 'what if' attached to it at all. This is the Aspen fear, and although it is irrational it is no less strong for that.

Fears of all kind lead naturally to worry, which can be a debilitating condition in its own right, not least because it so often leads to sleepless nights and stress. White Chestnut is the remedy for constant worry and oppressive, unwanted thoughts. For people who don't seem to have a care in the world but who go through mental torture inside, Agrimony is the remedy to choose.

As has been suggested, as far as possible it is a good idea for fathers-to-be to prepare for their new role as soon as possible. Human beings are not instinctive parents so there is a lot of learning to be done. For men one of the best places to start is at the local clinic where the mother-to-be will be attending her ante-natal classes. Most women like their partners to come with them and learn the basic relaxation and massage techniques that are used to help women through labour. Even if the man forgets everything he learns when the moment of truth arrives, the relationship between the couple and the sense that this is something they have to work at together will both have been strengthened. And at least he can offer emotional support and a hand to hold and be at her side all the time.

And of course this support is needed all through the pregnancy. The physical and emotional changes taking place in a woman as the pregnancy advances are major ones, and we men can really only guess at the difficulty involved in facing them. Although you cannot completely share these feelings you can at least try to help in an indirect way.

First of all, make allowances. Your partner may at times feel frustrated and angry at her inability to do things she once took for granted. This may lead her to take out her frustrations on you, and it can be hard not to react. You might tactfully suggest some flower remedies for her – such as Beech for intolerance of others and Cherry Plum for loss of control – but equally keep a watch on your own reactions. If you start sulking or fly into a tantrum you're not doing anyone any good. Take Willow for the first, Cherry Plum for the second.

Second, try to listen. Men are notoriously bad at talking about emotions, and many seem to think that a poor emotional life is something to be proud of. Don't be proud of it, change it, because if you don't try to understand and empathise with the way your wife is feeling you are not really taking part fully in the experience and you won't be as much help to her as you should be. If you have difficulty getting involved with her feelings, a number of the remedies might help, depending on your exact state of mind. Water Violet would help if you were holding yourself aloof from emotional involvement, for example, while Vine would be the remedy to temper a lack of compassion caused by your expecting others to think and act the way you want.

Third, learn what is going on. Considering the fact that every father today has had basic biology taught at school it is amazing how many men remain completely ignorant of the process of pregnancy and childbirth. If you take a little trouble to read a book on the subject and follow your partner's progress the whole thing will seem more real and at the same time less traumatic because you will know what to expect.

The fourth thing you can and should do is help with the arrangements for the day of the birth and for coming home afterwards. Not only will this take some of the strain off your partner but practical involvement will also help you to prepare emotionally for the new baby as well as reassuring your wife that you still love her and want the child as much as she does. Here are some ideas for the sort of things you can do:

- Help redecorate the house.
- Help choose the pram, the car seat, the carry cot and all the other extras.
- Help pack the bag your partner will take with her to the hospital.
- Help prepare the things the baby will need to come home in.
- Help plan travel arrangements on the day of the birth and accept responsibility for filling the petrol tank in the car, keeping spare change for the hospital car park and the phone, keeping the midwives' phone number by the phone and so on.
- Help to control visitors to the house (in the last few weeks before the birth and for weeks afterwards your partner will need rest, and over-enthusiastic friends and relations need to be rationed to short visits in ones and twos rather than mob-handed family excursions).

You might have noticed that each of these points begins with the word 'help'. This is because however anxious and nervy you are your partner is more so, because after all she is the one who is pregnant and she is the one who is doing the real work. If you start marching around assuming control you are asking for trouble. Your role in all of this should be that of a willing helper, then, and if you find it hard to play this role you should consider what remedy would be most appropriate for you – particular ones to consider might be Vine, Beech, Rock Water, Impatiens and Heather.

In the course of your reading about pregnancy you will have found out what labour is and how it starts. The first stage of labour is when the womb muscles contract so as to make room for the baby to emerge. When they start the contractions are few and far between and don't last very long, but over a period of time they get stronger and more frequent. You will have been advised by the hospital how frequent they should be before you phone in – it's usually when they are coming every ten minutes or so – but if you or your partner want reassurance there is no harm in phoning in at once. Make sure you have timed the frequency and duration of the last five or six contractions before you do so as the midwife will need this information to tell how far along the labour is. You will be glad now that you attended fathers' evening at the ante-natal class because you will know how to relieve the pain with pressure on the lower back, and you will be able to help your partner maintain control over her breathing. Rescue Remedy is a great help at this time as it can help overcome panic and faintness, and the inevitable physical and emotional shock that she (and you!) are going through.

At some time during this first stage there may be a 'show', the release from the vagina of a clot of blood and mucus. This is normal and nothing to worry about; and don't worry either if there doesn't seem to be one, since it can be very slight. The sac of liquid that surrounds the baby in the womb may also break at this time, although often this does not happen until much later. When the waters break or the show appears you should call the midwife: there is no danger, but either could be a sign that labour is advancing rapidly.

Do not be surprised or unduly put out if your partner pushes you away at some point during labour. There is a great deal of emotional energy and pain involved in giving birth and occasionally some of this is visited on the father's head simply because he is the nearest person available. In fact it is quite common for women close to the moment of birth to turn the air blue, and this is nothing to worry or get upset about: you would probably use some fairly ripe language yourself if you were going through what she is.

The first stage of labour can all be over inside two hours or it can go on for a couple of days. Before the end comes you will be packing up to go to the hospital. Your partner's bag, with a clean nightdress, maternity pads and so on will have been packed and ready some time before, as will some nappies and changing equipment for the new baby. If you haven't already packed a bag for yourself, here are a few of the things you might need to take with you:

- Change for parking meters, phone calls, vending machines etc.
- A list of all the people you want to call as soon as the baby is born.
- A credit card and a phonecard.
- A long, easy-to-read book.
- Nuts, fruit, biscuits or any other snack you or you partner might want in four or five hours' time.
- Some cold bottled mineral water and a flannel.
- A thermos flask full of coffee.
- Rescue Remedy and type remedies for you and your partner.

If you have taken care of the travel arrangements as suggested above you will not have to worry about the petrol station being closed, and the local taxi firm's number will be ready to hand just in case. You will also have rehearsed the trip to the maternity ward so that you know the way and know where to park and where the entrance to the hospital is. Thanks to this you should not have any trouble getting to the maternity ward long before the second stage of labour.

This begins when the mouth of the womb is fully dilated, and the whole stage is very short, usually lasting less than an hour. The midwife will help your partner into a comfortable birthing position and will help her to begin pushing in time with the contractions. This is very hard work. You can help by breathing with her and offering lots of encouragement and praise when she pushes. You can also help by putting your arm around her and helping to hold her sitting up. This makes it easier for her to push down and so helps speed things along. Your partner may also welcome the occasional cooling feel of a cool flannel laid on her forehead, and a few drops of Rescue Remedy can be added to the flannel before you apply it. Rescue Remedy can also be added to a glass of water which she can sip as the second stage proceeds.

Soon the top of the baby's head appears. Some men prefer not to look at this stage, and that is of course a personal choice. For myself, I was resolved not to look until the sheer wonder of what was happening made all my squeamishness vanish. Once the head is out the baby's body falls out very quickly, and there you are: a father.

WHEN THE BABY ARRIVES

When they first come out into the world babies are not like the pink, cuddly things in nappy commercials. They are usually dark red or purplish, blotchy and corrugated by being in fluid for so long, and often smeared in blood and vernix, a whitish substance that protects them in the womb. Their hands and feet may be white and puffy and their genitals swollen, so if you are not prepared for this you could be surprised and even alarmed, thinking that there might be something wrong. There isn't, and any swelling and puffiness soon disappear.

It's common nowadays for the new baby to be put on her mother's tummy as soon as she is born, but there are things to be checked and sometimes the midwife may forget to do this. You can always ask the midwife for the baby on your partner's behalf.

If you and your partner have been using Rescue Remedy during labour this can be continued now if it is needed. Some new parents may feel unsettled by what has happened and find that old associations and habits intrude into their thoughts even in the delivery room, and for this Walnut can be given. Walnut can also help the baby adjust to his new world – an adjustment that is of course much greater than the one his parents have to make since for him everything is strange and has to be learned from scratch. Instead of or as well as Walnut many practitioners advise giving Rescue Remedy to the new baby immediately after the birth to help him to cope with the shock and trauma of being born. Others suggest other remedies instead, often one of the five used in the composite Rescue Remedy such as Star of Bethlehem for shock, Clematis for faintness, Rock Rose for terror or Impatiens for undue agitation.

If the new mother has been taking any of these remedies herself, and if she is breast-feeding the baby, there is no need to give remedies to the baby separately. The beneficial effects will pass from mother to baby along with the mother's milk. If the baby is being fed with a bottle then a couple of drops of the selected remedy can be added to the bottle, or the baby's lips can be moistened with water to which the drops have been added.

The Bach Flower Remedies are of course completely safe and

have never been known to cause any adverse reaction in anyone of any age, but all the same two words of warning need to be given before you treat a small baby. Firstly, never give babies the drops undiluted from the stock bottles because they are preserved in pure brandy. Secondly, always consult the midwife or a doctor if you are in any doubt about your baby's health or well-being.

Birth and the early days of caring for the baby are without any doubt far tougher on the mother than on the father. As well as the pain and exhaustion caused by labour there may be stitches to recover from and sore and cracked nipples caused by the first attempts at breast-feeding. Unlike the father, who at first has the house to himself, the mother is from the start at the beck and call of the new baby, so that she gets little sleep just when she is at a low ebb anyway.

Olive is the remedy for tiredness and can usefully be given at this time, but tiredness is often not the only problem. Some women may take several weeks to build a bond fully with their babies, and their own lack of emotion may make them feel guilty and inadequate. Pine is a useful remedy at such times, helping to put feelings into perspective and stopping the new mother from blaming herself for things that are beyond her control. It has been estimated that as many as 80 per cent of women feel some degree of anxiety or mild depression after the birth, and Aspen and Mustard respectively would be an appropriate remedy for groundless feelings of fear and depression. Mustard could also be given to help the more serious condition known as post-natal depression. This is characterised by tearfulness and emotional outbursts, insomnia, loss of appetite and anxiety. It affects perhaps 10 per cent of mothers, and if you suspect your partner is suffering from it you should seek medical advice as soon as possible.

Although it might not seem so at the time the new father often needs help to maintain his emotional equilibrium as well. The chances are he will start off on a wave of euphoria and will be full of plans for the future and swept away by the desire to do the right thing by mother and baby alike. But just as likely he will feel confused and disorientated by the new demands placed upon him. He won't be able to come and go as he pleases any more. Simple things like listening to music or watching the television are made next to impossible because when the baby is asleep he mustn't be woken and when he is awake he must be tended to.

The birth of a baby represents a new stage in your life and in your personal growth. It's important then to be able to let go of the past and embrace the future. If you do the rewards are tremendous, but if you are held back from change by the clinging mists of your old way of life tremendous strain will be put on yourself and on your wife, who will be left quite literally holding the baby. Just as it could help in the early days, so Walnut is the first remedy to consider if you are having trouble making these necessary changes. You might also consider Honeysuckle where you find that you are thinking so much of the old freedoms that you are incapable of enjoying the deeper fulfilment of the present.

Other men who are anxious to be good fathers will feel guilt when career demands force them to take a back-seat role in the raising of their children. This problem is compounded by the fact that for a time at least the man will probably be the sole bread-winner and will often need to work longer hours in order to make up for the loss of his partner's earnings. If he tries to fit too much into the day then tiredness and stress are the inevitable results. Pine is the remedy for guilt, while for overwork Oak is one possible remedy, or Vervain where extra hours have been embraced with a little too much enthusiasm, perhaps as a way of showing what a good provider you can be. Olive is always a useful stop-gap where physical tiredness is a problem but, if possible, the underlying emotional cause should be treated as well, and this will usually be based on the person's type remedy.

Guilt can also be a problem where work comes to seem a refuge from the mess and noise of a young family, so that the father finds himself thinking up reasons to work late rather than return home and join in the bedtime marathon. Again, Pine can help bring a sense of fairness, balance and responsibility back while at the same time reducing the negative effects of guilt.

Other men seem unable to accept that their partners are no longer able to provide the spotless homes and punctual dinners they have come to expect. Such people might benefit from Beech, the remedy for those who are unfairly critical of other people. Chicory could also be a help in some cases: this is the remedy for people whose possessiveness leads them to interpret the smallest slight as evidence of neglect. A Chicory man is quite capable of seeing a cold dinner not as a sign that his partner has been struggling with a fractious baby all day, but as a deliberate snub. Ours is a possessive society, and it can be difficult suddenly having to share your partner with a demanding baby. Chicory is the remedy to soften possessive love into inclusive love, directed outward rather than focused on the Chicory person alone.

Other remedies that might come in useful as you get used to your new baby and the responsibilities she brings include:

- Centaury to help you be the father you want to be instead of the father your father (or mother) thinks you ought to be.
- Cerato if you lack confidence in your own judgement on the best way to love and care for your child.
- Cherry Plum when a screaming baby drives you to distraction so that you fear you might do something awful.
- Elm for the moments when the responsibility of bringing up a child seems too much to cope with.
- Impatiens if you feel frustrated when the baby gets in the way of the things you want to achieve.
- Red Chestnut for the fear that some awful accident or illness will affect the baby.
- Rock Water if you use parenthood as an excuse to become a martyr and give up pleasures unnecessarily.
- Vine if you tend to play the heavy-handed father and are too strict with your child.
- Water Violet if you find it hard to get emotionally involved with the business of parenting and tend to stay aloof and apart.

INFERTILITY

Most people assume that when they try to have a child they will not have to wait more than a few months to achieve their aim. After all, the underlying message of contraception is that it is all too easy to get someone pregnant without even meaning to. When the months go by without any sign of a pregnancy this can be very worrying, then, but it might be some comfort to know that you are not alone. After a year of trying as many as three couples out of 20 will have failed to conceive.

A man is said to be infertile when he has a low sperm count. The phrase 'low sperm count' is however rather misleading since what is being counted is not just the number of sperm in a given quantity of semen but also the amount of semen being produced, the proportion of sperm that is not fully functional and the degree of activity that the functional sperm display. Once a low sperm count has been discovered the actual cause of the low count will be sought. This may be some physical malformation such as a blockage that prevents the sperm reaching the penis, or a functional problem such as an infection or a hormone deficiency. Too much alcohol or coffee can also depress the sperm count, as can any number of psychological and environmental factors including depression and – strange but true – the wearing of tight trousers.

Different causes will lead to different treatments. Many of the physical defects may be corrected by surgery. Drug treatment can be used to correct the levels of chemicals in the body. And if the problem is down to the man's lifestyle he may be advised to cut down his intake of nicotine, alcohol and caffeine, and generally to eat better and take more exercise. Psychological and personal problems will be dealt with in an appropriate way. Finally, and if the problem cannot be resolved satisfactorily by other means, artificial insemination may be tried.

Basically there are two types of artificial insemination. Where the man is able to produce adequate sperm, perhaps after treatment of some kind, his own semen will be used if this is possible. If the sperm count is too low to make this a viable alternative then artificial insemination by donor – known from its initials as AID – may be recommended. This involves the fertilisation of the woman's egg with sperm donated by another man. The donor's identity is never known to the couple, nor does he learn who they are, and the resulting child is officially the child of the couple rather than the donor father. As far as possible the donor is usually chosen to resemble the father in terms of ethnic origin, height and so on to ensure that the child will not look too different from him.

Finally, and in cases where none of the above solutions is possible (or acceptable to the couple), then there may be the chance to adopt a child.

Properly speaking infertility is not a specifically male problem any more than it is a specifically female one: it is a problem shared by a couple. Nevertheless a man's reactions to infertility are often very different from his partner's. Whereas the woman is usually more prepared to acknowledge that there might be a problem for which she can get help, many men are reluctant to see doctors for any reason, still less one that is so intimately bound up with their self-image as 'real' men. There is a perceived stigma about infertility that leads some men to refuse to even consider the idea that a low sperm count might be the problem. And they may categorically refuse to consider testing even when it is demonstrated to them that men are as likely as women to suffer from reproductive disorders and that the matter has nothing to do with one's masculinity or the nature of one's sexuality. There may be an element of the negative Vine state in such behaviour, since it involves inflexibility and a wilful refusal to listen to people who know better.

Other men who shy away from such thoughts do so with a laugh, and try to make a joke of the whole thing. This refusal to take the possibility seriously can be infuriating for others, but it is no less painful for the man himself since the worries he represses during the day only return to haunt him at night. Agrimony is the remedy for such people. Men who blame themselves for being infertile may be helped by Pine, the remedy for guilty feelings, which will help them to remain positive about the problem and accept things without self-reproach.

The final route to fatherhood for people who cannot have their own children is to consider adoption – and there may of course be many other reasons to consider adoption as well, the simplest and best being the desire to give a child a good and loving home. Once it was fairly common for unmarried mothers to have their babies and put them up for adoption, since there were few alternatives apart from illegal abortion and ill-founded marriages, but things have changed. Nowadays, with the stigma of being a single parent removed (more or less), free, legal abortion and improved contraception, the smaller number of women who do go to full term are more likely to want to keep their children.

The start of the adoption process comes when you approach an agency. The main agencies in the UK are local Social Services Departments, but there are also private adoption agencies, some of them associated with particular religious groups, and some of them charging a fee for their services. Whichever agency you approach you will be screened thoroughly to ensure that you can offer a safe and loving home to the child. The system is rigorous and tough, as it has to be if it is to weed out child abusers and others who might do more harm than good to the children in their care. Although no-one could argue with this in theory, in practice the system makes it very difficult for anyone who is not part of a stable heterosexual relationship to adopt a child, and single men and male homosexual couples are the least likely to be successful. Nevertheless, some have managed it and have gone on to make excellent parents, and there is nothing to stop genuine people from these groups from applying and making their case.

Age can also be a problem if you are determined to adopt a baby rather than an older child. This is because there are more couples wanting to adopt babies than there are babies to go around, so that in order to restrict the number of people applying agencies only provide babies to younger couples. If you have delayed trying for a family until quite late in life you may find that your choice will be limited to toddlers or school-age children. If you are sure that you want a baby you may still be able to adopt a handicapped child or a baby born in another country.

Of course, adoption is a very serious business and if you are at all lukewarm about it you will be weeded out of the process in fairly short order. This does not mean however that you need to make up your mind irrevocably before you approach an agency. Indeed the best way to find out what you really want is to start the process off and get the help of professional, impartial assessors. You will not do your application any harm by appearing a little unsure of yourself at first, since agencies want to make sure you are committed to adoption for the right reasons and might actually be on their guard if you seem too gung-ho about things.

The agency's job is always to put the needs of the child first; and of course you will need to be able to do that too if you are to make a good father. There are so many emotions flying around during and after the adoption process, however, that it can be difficult to see what is best for anyone. And at times, when the way ahead is not clear, the Bach Flower Remedies can be a great help in restoring your clear-sightedness. This applies while you are waiting to adopt and even more so once your new child is settling into your home. For example:

- Clematis is the remedy to help when your dreams and ambitions for the future prevent you from dealing with the reality of the process you are going through, or when you withdraw from hard decisions into a never-never land.
- Beech will help if you feel critical and intolerant of other ways of life: the chances are that the child you eventually adopt will come from a background very different from yours and you will have to demonstrate to the agency that you can cope with this in a non-judgemental way.
- When the responsibility you are taking on feels too much for you, Elm is the remedy to select.
- For discouragement, try Gentian.
- For impatience with the slow progress you and the child are making, choose Impatiens.
- If you find that the searching enquiries made into your home life and your past undermine your confidence so that you no longer trust your own judgement and rely too much on other people's opinions, try Cerato.
- Larch is for you if you are convinced that whatever you decide it will end in failure.

These are just some of the remedies that might help. The actual remedies to choose in your case will depend on who you are and how you respond to the ups and downs of adoption. For more information on adoption and the whole adoption process, see Deborah Fowler's excellent book *A Guide to Adoption*, which is listed in the appendix.

PARENTING OLDER CHILDREN

As children grow up a great deal of maturity and flexibility is required of fathers. The rules that have helped the family run on an even keel up to now are suddenly all up for grabs. Every and any issue can create a storm, from a political opinion voiced in front of the nine o'clock news to the thorny question of how late a late night out should be. At such times it can be a useful exercise to think back to your own youth and how you used to feel when your parents carried on treating you as a child when it was obvious to you and your friends that you were already grown up and thinking for yourself.

Some men react to the challenges posed by their adolescent children by trying to clamp down even harder in an effort to recover their authority. Vine would help where this represents an effort to dominate over other lives or where discipline was carried to cruel extremes. For those men who are frightened that they will lose their children's affection if they let them stray too far from home, Chicory would be the remedy to soften the possessiveness that is poisoning their love. This is also the remedy to counteract self-serving attempts to impose high standards of behaviour and duty, perhaps learned in childhood but no longer appropriate for the present day. On the other hand, a taskmaster who acted from intolerance of other ways of life, rather than from the desire to control his loved ones, would need Beech rather than Chicory. Those who are frightened that something terrible will happen to their children if they are allowed to go off by themselves would benefit from Red Chestnut, since this would get things into perspective and allow sensible decisions to be made that allow the children to spread their wings safely and at the appropriate time of life.

Sometimes attempts to prevent children from growing up are founded on vanity. As adolescents mature and start making friends of the opposite sex, wearing the latest fashions and considering all kinds of exciting careers and educational opportunities it can hit poor old dad for the first time that the day of his generation really is coming to an end. If this leads to melancholy thoughts, Gentian is the remedy to banish them. Any tendency to try to live off past glories would need Honeysuckle.

More dramatic still is the father who tries to relive his past by going into competition with his children. He may flirt or start affairs in the effort to show that he still has what it takes. Or he may try to adopt the latest fashions himself, to the deep embarrassment of his children and his partner. He may think he is being bold and unconventional, but to others he will appear silly and immature. Different mental states may underlie his actions, of course, from the fear of getting older (Mimulus) and dislike of the way he looks now that he is older (Crab Apple) to a chronic lack of balance (Scleranthus), purposelessness (Wild Oat) and simple jealousy (Holly). Whatever the exact remedy or combination of remedies called for, the aim is the same, namely to help him see that he is still important and valuable in himself, and that instead of a vain effort to be a teenager again he could relax and enjoy the greater experience and maturity that his age and his experience have brought him.

While some men are jealous of their growing or grown-up children and want to be like them, others are scared that their children will be too much like they used to be. Remembering how they once criticised their fathers there must be some apprehension that they will suffer the same fate – worse, it might be justified. The father who finds it hard to put his point of view faced with the storms of adolescent virtue might benefit from Centaury. If he relies on brute force to win arguments then Vine might be more appropriate. Beech is the remedy for intolerance of other people's points of view and on many occasions would be equally helpful to both father and offspring.

An entirely different kind of feeling that can steal over a parent whose children are growing up too fast is nostalgia not for adolescent freedoms but for the joys of parenting young children. The father will hark back to the long-gone days when small, cuddly babies would coo and smile at him, or toddlers follow his every move and pronouncement with interest and open adulation. In contrast, boisterous, unpredictable and recalcitrant adolescents can seem very hard work indeed. Honeysuckle is of course the remedy for nostalgia when it gets in the way of enjoying today, while the man who grumbles all the time about the inevitable might need Willow for his lack of interest in his growing children and his tendency to speak unkindly and to think in a negative way. Chicory is once more the remedy for those who enjoyed being the focus of constant affection and feel deprived and slighted when it is withdrawn.

Of course dad is not always to blame and many of the problems fathers face in taking care of their adolescent sons and daughters can be laid fairly at the door of the children themselves. With a little thought, some consideration, and moderate strength of will, most problems will not be too serious however. Perhaps the most important balance to strike is between giving teenagers freedom to explore who they are and find their feet in the world while at the same time keeping some control. It's all too easy to go too far in one direction or another, and either give no guidance at all or try to dictate every move regardless of what the children themselves want. The danger of no control is that teenagers will see it as a sign that you do not care enough to take trouble over them. However strong and independent they may claim (or appear) to be they will be very unsure of themselves and your regard for them if they do not have a definite, concerned parent to kick against. On the other hand too much control will antagonise them and can create a very unpleasant atmosphere for years to come.

The remedies might help you at this juncture. For example:

- If you avoid confrontation and are happy to let things drift, adopting a fatalistic attitude, then Wild Rose is the remedy to select.
- If you do not face up to your children directly but grumble and complain about them behind their backs then Willow would be the remedy to choose.
- Heather would be a better choice if you talk to all and sundry about what is wrong with your children but are incapable of listening to what the children themselves think.

- The doormat father who puts up no resistance to his children's demands is in need of Centaury.
- The normally competent man who is overwhelmed and made to feel inadequate needs Elm.
- For the authoritarian father Vine is the remedy to counteract the tendency to dominate and ride roughshod over the needs of other people.
- A more subtle form of authoritarianism is shown by the Chicory father, who manipulates instead of commanding but is just as good at getting his own way without allowing the teenager freedom to make his or her own mistakes and learn from them.
- Beech is the remedy for intolerance of youth and its beliefs and opinions.
- The man who tries to be a strong example to his children but who is actually too wrapped up in perfecting himself to give real guidance would benefit from Rock Water.

The ideal solution to the problem of relationships between adults and growing children is to negotiate and agree with them what the limits on their behaviour will be. As with any negotiation you will probably not get everything you want, but you will get some of it, and because the limits have been agreed between you it will be easier for you to enforce them when they are transgressed. You are also showing your adolescent child that you appreciate the fact that she or he is older and more grown up now, as well as providing useful education in the very adult art of compromise. Your aim then is to remain calm and in control of yourself, and emotionally balanced so that you can provide love, comfort, and security and say what you really think openly and honestly – and then not feel so threatened that you cannot learn from the honest answers you get in return. In truth few if any parents ever manage to be like this all of the time – but almost every parent can learn to be like this enough of the time to make a difference, and the remedies can help you achieve that reasonable goal.

Finally, this is a good place to mention the dangers of trying to get your children to live the life you would have liked, in retrospect, to lead yourself. Your growing adults (because that's the way you now need to think of them) must be allowed to choose their own interests and careers even if they do not fit in with your ambitions or family traditions. If you try to stop them making their own choices you will either fail and make yourself unnecessarily miserable, or you will succeed and put them on the road to eventual failure and disappointment, not to mention stunting their ability to make their own choices in the future.

Children who might be unduly influenced by selfish parents into following a course that doesn't suit them might be helped by Centaury, which is the remedy for those who find it hard to say no to other people. Walnut is the remedy to help overcome the opinions and conventions embraced by other people when these hold them back from following their dreams. If the way ahead is not clear enough to start to formulate plans even then Wild Oat is the remedy to help them come to correct decisions about which path to take in life.

CHAPTER 6

THE SEARCH
FOR FULFILMENT

THE MID-LIFE CRISIS

The two great icons of the Western world are youth and success. You can be successful without being young or young without being successful. But if you are getting older without having achieved all the things you once dreamed of then you are a failure and you are running out of time. Judging by the depression, resentment, self-loathing, apathy and anxiety that many men feel as they approach their middle years this simple equation is widely accepted. Small wonder then that Derek Llewellyn-Jones can write in his book *Every Man* that 'many men in their middle years, between the ages of 40 and 65, are not in emotional balance.'

This lack of emotional balance at or around a man's fortieth or fiftieth birthday is often referred to as a 'male menopause'. In one way this description is apt, since middle-aged men in crisis can display many of the symptoms that are found in menopausal women, including tiredness, nervous tension and irritability. There is however a major difference between the true menopause and the male version. In women these changes have direct and obvious physical causes, in that the hormones that have controlled the reproductive cycle since adolescence begin to disappear until they become infertile when they are no longer producing eggs. Men are biologically capable of fathering children until the day they die, and the hormonal changes that they do experience tend to come in old rather than middle age. The symptoms of the male menopause, then, are entirely due to psychological or emotional disturbance. The physical changes associated with middle-aged men – such as the tendency to put on weight around the tummy, greying and thinning hair and a general loss of muscle and skin tone – do not themselves cause any hormonal changes that might explain the psychological effects. What they do, of course, is contribute to the feeling that one is getting older and running out of time.

The menopausal man is not struggling to adapt to a different chemical balance in his body. Instead he is trying to come to terms with what he has become. More, he is trying to bridge the gap between the reality of his modest successes and increasing years and the fantasy of everlasting vigour, youth, success and sexuality that is the prevailing Western myth of the male. His thoughts are turning probably for the first time to the fact that he is mortal. And it should not be forgotten that one of the reasons men do all these things at this time is that they are expected to do so. One of the ways society overvalues youth is by getting middle aged men to feel that they are already old. It is interesting to learn that in Japan, where youth is not valued so highly and only those who have turned fifty are considered fully mature, the symptoms we associate with the menopause are largely absent even in women.

The degree of pressure brought to bear on middle-aged men is demonstrated by the personality changes that can occur, with wild mood swings and a tendency to lose their temper at the least provo-cation. The fact that the menopausal man's wife is quite likely to be going through the climacteric at about the same time only serves to increase the tension. Both partners will need support and under-standing at a time when neither of them is best placed to provide it. And, as if all this was not enough for the poor male, this is also the time when children are going through adolescence, questioning all his values and assumptions and beliefs. And eventually they leave home, so that he and his partner are left to try to create a new centre for their diminished family, alone together for the first time in decades.

Because an individual's emotional state is the single and entire cause of the problems associated with the mid-life crisis the Bach Flower Remedies are particularly well placed to help. The following remedies are among those that would most often be considered for the menopausal man:

- Walnut for people who need help to make changes and break old unwanted links to ways of life that are now past.
- Hornbeam for those who cannot face the thought of the day ahead and their old routine.
- Agrimony for those men who laugh off their troubles or attempt to drown them in good living.
- Larch for loss of confidence.
- Elm for those who feel overwhelmed by their responsibilities.
- Wild Oat for those who are dissatisfied at not being able to find a worthwhile and fulfilling role in life.
- Willow for those who feel resentful against partners or other people who seem to be doing better than they are.
- Mimulus for the fear of getting older or of death (Aspen might also be used where the fear of death was a vague, superstitious dread rather than a rational fear).
- Mustard for black depressions that descend apparently without cause.
- Gorse for despair, depression and hopelessness that are associated with a particular, named situation or thought.
- Scleranthus for general indecision and mood swings.
- Wild Rose for apathy and the feeling that nothing is worth doing.
- Cherry Plum for loss of control and violent or suicidal impulses.
- Crab Apple for the man who dislikes or is disgusted by his own appearance and physical condition.
- Oak for the man who tries to ignore the crisis and plod on with his everyday work, often extending himself beyond the point of breakdown.
- Chicory for those who miss being surrounded by love and attention when children leave home.
- Beech for those who are intolerant of their partners or their children and their ways of thinking.

However, the mid-life crisis should be seen as more than a series of emotional problems that need to be righted so that the man can resume his former course. The point of using the Bach Flower

Remedies on these occasions is not to squeeze the discontented man back into his mould so that he can go on changeless unto death. Still less is it to keep him quiet so that he won't embarrass his children, or to set his sense of helplessness into concrete so that his failure makes youth shine the brighter. The real aim is in every case to restore his sense of balance and get rid of the negative states that might prevent him from seeing where he really wants to go. The remedies always work to help people be themselves and take control so that they can grow and develop in the ways they choose. Instead of approaching it as an imposition or the beginning of the end, then, you can take control of your mid-life crisis and turn it into an opportunity. It is to this possibility that we now turn.

CHANGING COURSE

It is obvious – or should be – that ageing is a natural process you can't do anything about. You need to adapt to getting older. You cannot regain your lost youth or have your time again and it is a waste of time trying to do so. This is common advice in the literature of middle and old age, but all too often the answer to the restlessness of mid-life is simply to get yourself in order, give up your dreams, knuckle down and start saving for retirement. That is not enough.

Middle age is not just a pause before old age, but rather the start of a long period of maturity. It is a time in which you can accomplish twice as much as you did before. Your children will be older and in many cases already living away from home, and you are probably less inclined to work all hours of the day and night than you were when you were younger. Finances tend to be more secure than they were so there is less need to chase money at all costs. This leaves you more time than ever before to think about yourself and the things you need.

In the previous 40 or 50 years you have been involved on and off in examining who you are and defining and redefining what is really important to you. You have been working to achieve your dreams of personal fulfilment and happiness, building family relationships with your children and your partner, and at times taking risks by changing the whole course of your life. You may not have been very conscious of this process but you have still put a lot of work into it. Why on earth should you even consider stopping these activities now, with all your experience and all your accumulated knowledge about the world and your place in it? Why stop when for the first time in years you have the time and security to make real changes? Why stop precisely at the time when society is practically demanding that you take a good look at yourself?

You should not consider stopping, of course. But not stopping does not mean throwing everything away or indulging in escapist behaviour of a destructive or trivial sort. For example, everyone knows of someone who has suddenly abandoned his wife of many years to take up with a much younger woman. For a few people this is the right thing to do, when the original relationship has broken down irretrievably and where the new couple are genuinely in love. But in many cases the attempt to recapture young love may achieve little more than proving a point, showing that you can still do it – whatever it is. Other men don't leave their families but indulge in affairs, with the same lack of real results. These are destructive attempts at making things better because they do not address the real issues: they encourage you to run away from who you are rather than helping you change and grow. In other words, if your relationships are not satisfactory you will not find much improvement if you take the same set of expectations and simply transfer them onto someone else. This is a variation on the Chestnut Bud state, where you repeat the same basic mistakes over and over and are unable to learn from your experiences. What you need to do is learn the lessons of your life and face up to any emotional problems that may be working against your happiness. Then if a change has to be made you can at least make it with some hope of success.

If apathy and resignation are not the answers, then, and sudden change is often unpremeditated and counter-productive, what avenues to change are left?

All of us carry around a set of assumptions that we base all our conscious decisions on. They are the things we take for granted, much as we take for granted the sun rising in the morning and the stars coming out at night. They seem so obvious to us that we rarely question them or ask ourselves if experience shows them to be true. For example, some men go every morning to jobs they hate because of the money they make. The money doesn't make them happy yet they still go in. The idea that they might be happier with less money if they had more time at home or a more satisfying job is dismissed out of hand or, more often, never considered. This is because there is a common assumption in our society that men should earn more each year, and that accepting a job for less money is only ever done when there is no other choice but to do so. Others are locked into self-abuse through drink or overeating but put off doing anything about it because they are too busy or under too much stress at the moment. The assumption here is that there will always be a tomorrow when the diet can begin and the drinking stop. Others still assume that they and their partners are the same people that they were when they married twenty or thirty years before, and that for this reason there is no point in trying to change the nature of the relationship.

Before you can make sensible changes in your life you need to examine these assumptions. The key is to look at the areas of your life that you are unhappy with and root out the attitudes that allow the unhappiness to persist. For men this often means trying once again to cope with the expression of emotions and overturning the stereotypical role of leader, provider and authoritarian. It means learning how to touch and be touched, especially if you think you don't need to. It means learning to listen to other people's arguments instead of looking always for a way of winning at all costs. It means learning how to measure success as fulfilment and happiness rather than by the size of a car or the weight of a bank balance. These things are difficult and take time and commitment to achieve. The remedies can help to keep you on an even keel when you are faced with difficult, uncertain feelings and emotions along the way.

For example, if the thought of making some change or other leaves you anxious or afraid then Mimulus is the first remedy to consider. For the vaguer feelings of unease and fear that are not centred on a known, named cause, Aspen is the remedy to choose, while if you are scared of the effect the new you will have on your family then Red Chestnut should be selected instead. If you are uncertain whether or not to do something then Scleranthus is the remedy to choose, while you should try Cerato if you know what you want but lack confidence in your own judgement.

Inevitably, when you question your own assumptions about yourself you will be questioning your relationships with your family. Your partner in particular may feel threatened by this. This is because as a couple you long ago came to an arrangement that would allow you to get along together. You both had to give a bit to do this, sacrificing freedoms and desires in order to achieve a workable compromise. If you now decide that you want things to be different you are in effect saying that the agreement has to be negotiated again from scratch. Unless your partner feels the same she will probably feel threatened and try to maintain the status quo. You may need the help of Centaury if you find yourself being dominated and led along by unreasonable demands. If your partner's reaction – real or assumed – leaves you feeling guilty then Pine is the remedy to help you see things clearly and act the way that is right in the long run for you and your family.

On the other hand, it is just as likely to be your partner who wants change while you try to hold her back and keep things as they were. For example, some men become manipulative when their partners after years of child rearing announce that they want to go back to work. Often this is a Chicory state, since the real fear is that she won't be giving all her attention and love to you any more. Other men may fly into rages or get into a temper at the slightest provocation – Cherry Plum is the remedy for the loss of emotional control, while Holly is for the anger that is based on hatred, jealousy or suspicion. You may resent the fact that your partner is suddenly so independent when other women (or so it seems in the adverts on television) are content to sit at home and look after their husbands. Willow is the remedy to stop you feeling sorry for yourself and be rather more generous in your feelings.

Apart from relationships, probably the biggest source of mid-life crisis is work. Like those women who dread turning into their mothers, many men hate the idea that they might turn into replicas of their first bosses, those colourless men with their out-of-date ideas and stick-in-the-mud ways. It can be very hard to discover that you yourself are no longer seen by your bosses as a bright young man with a future, but as a steady, reliable and rather unadventurous old hand. This is of course social stereotyping, since there is no reason why men over forty should not continue to be iconoclastic and full of ideas. Look at the careers of Picasso and Freud if you think this is not true. But the pressure is on people to conform, and many buckle down and do so.

Even worse is the feeling that you are not even in the right job. In adolescence most of us have ideas of how we want to earn our living, but inevitably very few ever achieve the careers, the success and the fame they wanted. For most, a career is a means to an end, but it still takes up five days out of seven and makes huge demands on energy and commitment. Mid-life doubts and regrets about the way things have turned out can lead to depression (Gentian or Gorse) and feelings of helplessness and apathy (Wild Rose). And however much you decide you want to change you might feel that you are trapped in your job due to economic and social pressures – the need to pay the mortgage, the need to support a family and the difficulty older men can have in finding alternative employment anyway. Coupled with this there may be regret or guilt at not having played a more active role in raising children (Honeysuckle or Pine) and resentment at the social pressures and the job that made this happen (Willow).

The key to resolving this crisis lies, as we suggested earlier, in a close look at your assumptions. Ask yourself the following questions and don't be satisfied with the first answer that comes to mind:

- Why do I want to work? Most people would automatically say that they go to work to make money, but there are all kinds of other factors that may be more important to you, such as status, companionship, the respect of your peers, achievement, or simply a love of routine. Having found the reasons you want to work you are in a better position to see how far your current career satisfies them and what changes would make you happier.

- Why did I end up in this job? You may have made a conscious decision and taken a lot of trouble and time to get to where you are now; or you may have just drifted into your job because it was the first thing that came along. There may be other hidden reasons too, such as choosing a particular career to please (or displease) a parent. If you change jobs, will it be for the same, or for better reasons?

- What do I love/hate most about this job? You may be surprised at how little there really is to complain about, in which case you might look elsewhere in your life for the cause of your discontent. Or you may be amazed that you have stuck it out so long. In any case you need to know what you do and don't like so that you can avoid the classic Chestnut Bud mistake of leaving a job because you don't like teamwork and stress only to take another job where you are working under stress in a team.

- How much do I know about my ideal career? It's all too easy to romanticise a job when you don't have to do it: that's why all the eulogising over manual labour is done by people who don't know one end of a shovel from another. If you are nurturing some secret ambition why haven't you tried it out yet, just to see if it fits your fantasy?

Just like the man who leaves his partner on a whim and regrets it ever afterwards, many men jump from one career to another without examining their motivations. All too often such moves turn out to be expensive and futile exercises in which one set of frustrations and unhappiness is exchanged for another. By taking the time to define what exactly makes you unhappy about your present situation you are better placed to make sensible, effective changes. This does not necessarily mean that other people will think they are sensible, but what other people think is really not the issue. Even the maddest career change is right if it is right for the person concerned.

By using the Bach Flower Remedies to help you through this and the other crises of middle age you will be better able to know your own mind. Far from being a conservative therapy which always brings you back to where you are and restricts change, the remedies are a means to self-knowledge and clear-sightedness. Both qualities are essential if a change of any kind is to be successful.

RELIGION AND BELIEF

Most of us most of the time go through life without seriously questioning who we are and what our place in the scheme of things really is. We accept, more or less, our religion (or lack of religion) but do not let it change our lives too much. We are absorbed in the daily routine of our lives and give little weight to higher purposes. When we are sad we cry and we laugh when we are happy, but we omit to consider that either happiness or sadness might have some deeper or higher purpose.

Nevertheless, almost everyone at one time or another will go through a crisis of belief of some sort. Of the male half of the species middle-aged and very young men are most prone to them, but they can occur at any age and take many different forms. For one man it will be a bereavement that will shake his faith in a loving God; for another some striking piece of hypocrisy on the part of a political leader will leave him questioning principles that have until now been the main planks of his moral system; for a third a simple sense of hopelessness will strike as if from nowhere so that the world seems a place of ashes and dirt in which nothing good can ever exist. And of course it can be just as distressing for a convinced atheist to witness a miracle.

How we react to our crises of belief depends on the kind of people we are. When negative emotions and characteristics are released by the crisis then the Bach Flower Remedies can help to turn the mind in a positive direction once more, so allowing the personality to grow and benefit from the crisis instead of being frozen by it. For example:

- Where the loss of certainty in your life leaves you struggling to find something worth doing, select Wild Oat.
- If you feel hot anger and hatred for those you now think have deceived you all this time, select Holly.

- When you sink into self-pity and take perverse delight in puncturing the contentment of others without trying to improve your own situation, select Willow.
- If you cling stubbornly to your ideas even though they have been fatally challenged, and are prepared to martyr yourself and your happiness to preserve your beliefs, select Rock Water.
- If the loss of your faith leaves you feeling black, ultimate despair as if you and your world are entirely destroyed, select Sweet Chestnut.
- If you begin to drift aimlessly and without purpose, becoming lethargic and mentally deadened, select Wild Rose.

The remedies can do even more at this difficult time. This is because they represent in themselves a simple and straightforward link to nature and the ordinary beauties of life. They are made from simple, unremarkable plants found growing wild and without human interference. The petals and leaves are floated in pure water and in many cases the action of the strong summer sun is all that is required to transfer their healing properties to the water. Everything about them is rooted in simplicity, just as Dr Bach himself wanted.

When life seems to have lost or changed its purpose this gentle echo of simple things can be a timely reminder that some things are intrinsically good and fine. After all, simple things often provide the greatest pleasures. Listing them can remind you of the ropes that attach you to the world. On my own list I would include watching my daughters Alex and Maddie talk and smile, sharing summer evenings, autumn walks and winter fires with my wife, Italian food, red wine and cold beer, the last verse of Eliot's *Prufrock*, the last passage in Joyce's *Dubliners*, Mozart's *Requiem* and the guitar solo in Led Zeppelin's *Since I've Been Loving You*. Your list would doubtless be different, which is as it should be. What matters is that the items on it can provide a bedrock when times get tough, a reliable foundation on which to rebuild your bridge to the rest of the doubtful universe.

Simplicity should not be confused with simple-mindedness, and this is not an attempt to discount the very real anguish that the loss of a belief or value system can bring. But in many, if not all cases, the problem is rooted in vanity, by which I mean the belief that you can do or ought to be able to understand everything. In fact you can't and you don't, and there's no reason at all to believe that the universe could ever be small enough to fit inside your ideas. If you could lose yesterday's certainties so quickly then there is every reason to think that today's are just as vulnerable. The truth is that you have to stand somewhere to see the rest of the world, but you can never see the place where you are standing. If you move somewhere else you can see where you were – that's why the flaws in your former beliefs are so obvious to you now – but now you can't see the place you have moved to. This means that however many moves you make – however many different places you find to stand – you do not and will not ever in this life know ultimate truth.

But you can still make the world better and richer for your presence and find joy in your existence. This is a small and simple truth, you see, but none the worse for that.

The same consciousness of our own fallibility might also serve as a gentle reminder to those who fervently embrace a new belief, a new political creed or the latest philosophy. In some cases these will be Vervain people taking their commitment to extremes and determined to convert the world. In others they will be Rock Water types, not concerned to convert others directly but rather seeking their own salvation first and so trying to impress by virtue of example rather than force of argument. Others still will be Beech people, intolerant of any system that isn't the same as theirs. All three types can at times become deaf to other ways of thinking and being. The Vervain, Rock Water or Beech remedies are given as appropriate to help encourage tolerance and understanding of other points of view and of people's – or our own – weaknesses. This is an important part of Dr Bach's lesson: a positive understanding of others and of ourselves and of our emotions, and a willingness to live with and learn from all three. This may be a simple principle to live by but it demands as much courage and honesty as any, and the potential rewards are great.

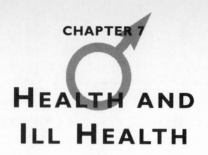

HEALTH AND
ILL HEALTH

MAINTAINING A HEALTHY LIFESTYLE

Whether it is a result of their upbringing or an inherited tendency to take more risks, men as a whole tend to pay a great deal less attention to their health than women do. In particular, men:

- Smoke more than women.
- Eat more animal fat.
- Drink more alcohol.
- Are less weight-conscious.
- Go to the doctor less often.

This last point is particularly interesting. It seems that men are reluctant to admit they need help with their health. Some of them are of course genuine Oak types who try to struggle on with their duties as if nothing is wrong. But for most men, regardless of their type, the problem is one of perception. It's as if it isn't quite the manly thing to take care of yourself. Whether they are Oaks or not, then, the result is often the same: by the time they do seek help it is rather later than it should be, and conditions which could have been cured relatively easily earlier on have had time to get established and are therefore harder to treat.

This is a great shame. Men are just as likely as women to fall ill and suffer from the effects of an unhealthy lifestyle, and are more likely to lead one. They are also prone to a range of diseases, from acne to Duchenne Muscular Dystrophy, which are largely confined to males. Fortunately it is relatively simple to improve things by taking a little thought (and a little time) to look at the way you live. In particular, there are five main, interrelated areas that you can work on: smoking, weight control, diet, exercise, and emotional health.

Since smoking and obesity will not apply to all men (some men do not smoke and others will never have a weight problem) they are dealt with later on in this chapter when we come to look at specific health problems. The other three are somewhat different since they are ingredients of a healthy lifestyle that all men at all times can plan into their lives. So diet, exercise and emotional health will be considered here.

The need to follow a sensible diet is probably accepted by most people, although men, in particular, are inclined to excuse their failure to do so on the grounds that the experts never agree on what a sensible diet is. It is true of course that there have been occasional and well-publicised reverses of policy towards specific foodstuffs. Once we were told to 'go to work on an egg', for example, but now we are advised to ration the number eaten in a week. Despite this, and despite the use the food industry makes of such disagreements to continue to sell unhealthy food, most experts do in fact agree on the fundamentals of a good diet. The main points are probably well known to most people already:

- Eat more fibre, such as fruit, (some) breakfast cereals, wholewheat bread and vegetables.
- Avoid processed foods.
- Eat less red meat.
- Eat more uncooked fruit and vegetables.
- Cut down on sugar and fat, especially animal fat.
- Cut down on dairy products and eggs, which are high in cholesterol.
- Eat more fish, especially oily fish.
- Grill food instead of frying it.

There are variations on this basic list. Some will eat fish but no animal or bird meat. Others will turn vegetarian and others still become strict vegans and refuse to eat any animal products at all including cheese and butter. Often there is a moral element in such decisions which can be as important or more important than any health consideration. And it is, of course, perfectly possible to be a vegan and still get all the vitamins, minerals and proteins you need from your normal diet – although it is fair to say it will take a little planning and thought to achieve this.

Additives are a particular cause of concern to many people. The idea of adding things to food in order to make it keep longer or make it look or taste more appealing is as old as salt beef and the spice trade. The difference today is that many of the additives being used are not natural products at all but artificial ones created in a laboratory. Even those that are natural are sometimes strange substances that have little or no nutritional value and would not even be called edible normally.

The food industry claims that additives as a whole are useful and necessary. But it is hard to see what real benefits artificial sweeteners such as Aspartame and Saccharin confer beyond the ability to continue unhealthy eating habits without putting on weight. You might be right to think that there is something obscene in the idea of calorie-free food in a world where so many suffer hunger and starvation: what in the end is the difference between this and a rich Roman vomiting during a feast so as to be able to eat more? As for food colouring like Tartrazine and Sunset Yellow, both have been linked to hyperactivity and emotional disturbances in young children. In fact particular groups of people can be allergic to almost any of the food additives commonly found on the supermarket shelf.

There are any number of reasons to be careful of what you eat. For a start you will find it much easier to maintain your normal weight if you eat sensibly. You will avoid many common health problems (some of which will be covered in full later in this chapter) such as heart disease, high blood pressure, constipation and a whole range of digestive problems. You will also feel more energetic and in control of your body and mind, not least because you will be introducing a vital area of simplicity into your everyday routine. The aesthetic improvement alone will enhance the quality of your life.

While you are thinking about what you eat, take some time to think about what you drink as well. Only recently the UK government raised the recommended safe level of alcohol consumption from 21 units a week (a unit being half a pint of beer, a single measure of spirits or a glass of wine) to 28 units. Medical opinion on the wisdom of this move is divided, but in any case if you are drinking substantially more than this on a regular basis there is no doubt that you are doing yourself long-term harm. For those with a serious alcohol problem there is more detailed information further on in this chapter.

The extra energy you gain when you follow a sensible diet will be a help when you start taking exercise. This is of course an essential part of a sensible weight reduction programme, but the benefits do not by any means stop there. Regular exercise tones up the body, reduces the risk of disease, strengthens the immune system and has positive psychological effects as well, leaving us not only healthier but happier about ourselves and our place in the world.

Exercise does not have to be violent to be beneficial, nor does it have to be prolonged. Unless you are already very fit, three 20 minute sessions a week of gentle jogging or swimming, or even a good brisk walk, will do as much good as an hour a day punishing yourself on the squash court – and you will be less likely to injure yourself in the process. The aim is to speed up the pulse a little and be just a little out of breath. Once your regime is no longer doing that, you can increase the amount you do a little at a time. But be sure to get the right equipment and train sensibly, or you run the risk of making yourself worse rather than better (see the entry on Sports Injuries later on in this chapter). And if you are more than 40 years old, a heavy smoker, seriously overweight or suffer from a respiratory or heart complaint, you should get the advice of a doctor before you start.

Probably the hardest thing about exercising is getting a routine established. For the first few sessions you will probably come up with any number of excuses why you could or should delay things. If you find yourself putting off getting started you might benefit from Hornbeam, the remedy for those who procrastinate and find it hard to get going. If you are convinced you will not be a success at exercising and that is your excuse for not getting on with things then

Larch would be the remedy to choose. And if you find yourself talking a great deal about exercise and eliciting everyone else's opinions on it without actually ever doing any then Cerato might help you to trust and abide by your decision to get fit irrespective of what others say.

But there are other reasons why people – especially not very healthy people – are reluctant to take the plunge. Standing in your new tracksuit and running shoes and looking at yourself in the mirror you may be frightened that younger more athletic people will laugh at you as you puff your way around the park. Or perhaps you are frightened of being chased by dogs or of being mugged. Mimulus is the remedy to counteract these fears, just as it is appropriate for those people who are shy and self-conscious by nature and so nervous of appearing in public in anything other than ordinary street clothes.

Once you have been exercising for a while there are other times when the Bach Flower Remedies might come in useful. If you have to miss a few sessions and take to blaming yourself for this, or if you castigate yourself for not making enough progress, then Pine could help to ease your tendency towards self-reproach. If you find yourself getting carried away by the exercise fad to such an extent that it is no longer a pleasure but a grim road to martyrdom, then Rock Water is the remedy to bring things back into perspective and remind you that you are exercising to improve the quality of your life, not to deny yourself pleasure. Vervain might help for a similar state of mind, where enthusiasm for the cause leads you to overdo things beyond your body's ability to cope, or even spend all your energy trying to persuade everyone else to join in. Those people who also do too much, but through endurance rather than enthusiasm, would be helped by Oak.

Many of the considerations and mental states catalogued above will also apply to the man who experiences problems sticking to a sensible diet. The remedies would be chosen using the same principles, as for example:

- Rock Water for the man who tries to set himself up as an example to others by following a particularly strict diet.

- Vervain for the man who passionately tries to convert everyone to the benefits of this or that regime.
- Chestnut Bud for the man who continually goes back to his former eating habits and is always trotting out the same excuses for doing so.
- Heather for the man who becomes so obsessed with what he is or isn't eating that he bores everyone he knows with the details.
- Gentian for the man who eats badly one day and is discouraged for days afterwards.

The aim of the Bach Flower Remedies is of course to promote and maintain mental and emotional health not just when it comes to exercise and diet but in all situations and stages of life. Having read this far in the book you should be in little doubt of the supreme importance of this, especially when it comes to facing disease. A sound mind, free from unnecessary worry and useless and trivial baggage, is able to direct its energy to fight disease effectively. Positive thinking and emotional health give you a head start whenever you are faced with a specific physical problem. As you will see in the rest of this chapter the remedies given to people suffering from physical complaints are always aimed at removing the negative thoughts that can stand in the way of the body's natural good health.

The remedies are not the only way to stay emotionally healthy. First, it is important to be in a web of good relationships of one kind or another. These can be centred on family or friends, but in all cases they need to be based on honesty and trust. It is also important to have reasons to want to go on living and keep on doing things since these will give you the resolve to keep fighting that you may need in particularly grave situations. And, above all, you need balance in your life: extremes of any kind, whether of apathy or effort, of luxury or frugality, will in the end do more harm than good. In the end the best friend you can have in your fight to be well is your own well-rounded and unfragmented spirit.

SPECIFIC PROBLEMS

Even if you do your best to stay healthy you will still fall ill from time to time. In illness as in health the Bach Flower Remedies can provide the support you need to keep to your own path even when ill health threatens to blow you off course. Every individual will react differently to different problems, of course, and for this reason selecting a remedy or remedies must always be done on an individual basis. Nevertheless, it can be a help to get some real suggestions that are related to specific problems. In this section, a number of health problems that are particularly associated with men are listed, along with some suggestions as to how the Bach Flower Remedies might help.

The principles according to which remedy selection is made will of course apply equally well to other health problems, from the simplest cold to the most dangerous of life-threatening diseases.

ACNE

Acne is particularly associated with young men. It usually starts in puberty, when rising hormone levels increase the amount of sebum being produced, blocking pores in the skin and leading to spots, pimples, blackheads and boils. These are usually found on the face and back. In severe cases acne can cause permanent scarring, and it may continue until the victim is in his twenties or thirties.

On a physical level there are three approaches to alleviating acne. The first is to try to keep the skin as clean as possible. There are a number of proprietary cleaning preparations that can be used to keep the pores clean, all of which may be obtained from chemists. You could also try treating the skin with Crab Apple, the cleansing remedy. To do this, add two drops of the remedy to a small amount of water and dab gently onto the affected areas with clean cotton wool. This is best done on a regular basis – morning and night, for example, and immediately after your normal cleaning routine.

The second physical approach to acne revolves around diet, and works on the theory that sugary and fatty foods like chocolate, sweets, chips and crisps make the condition worse. Fruit and fresh vegetables can be substituted for these suspect foods, and will also help by providing the essential vitamins skin needs to stay supple and healthy. For the same reason it is also a very good idea to try to drink around eight glasses of fresh mineral water every day. Alternatively, tea and coffee are better than nothing – but both can increase urination so they are not as good as water.

The last of the physical approaches involves the use of prescription drugs. Antibiotics are by far the commonest drugs given to people whose condition is bad enough to send them to a doctor. Usually this involves a high initial dose followed by about six months on a reduced dosage. For really severe cases of acne, where a skin specialist has been consulted, there may be treatment by a strong drug called isotretinoin, which works by cutting down the production of sebum and the bacteria level on the skin. Unfortunately there are side-effects associated with its use, including hair loss and conjunctivitis. It should be stressed though that most cases of acne are nowhere near serious enough to warrant the use of isotretinoin, which is very much a last resort.

The psychological effects of acne can be even greater than the physical effects, especially given the fact that it usually strikes young men just when they are beginning to become interested in sex and in their own personal attractiveness. The Bach Flower Remedies are of course ideally placed to help the individual deal with this aspect of the problem and so maintain a positive attitude towards getting well. Particular remedies that might be useful include:

- Crab Apple taken internally to cleanse the body and remove any feelings of self-dislike caused by the condition.
- Larch for any loss of confidence.
- Gorse for a feeling of hopelessness.
- Mimulus for fear that the condition will worsen, fear of ridicule, fear of social occasions and so on.
- Willow for bitterness and self-pity.
- Impatiens for frustration at the slowness of a cure.
- Agrimony for mental torture hidden behind a smile.
- Oak for the youth who tries to go on as normal but is being worn down by the problem.
- Wild Rose for apathy and resignation, as in the case of the

youth who says: 'I might as well eat a bag of chips and forget about washing because it's not going to get better.'

It is believed that stress and anxiety can make acne worse so efforts should be made to keep worries and fears under control. White Chestnut is the remedy for continual worrying thoughts; Impatiens and Vervain can help those who in their different ways put themselves under stress. Mimulus and Aspen are the usual remedies for anxiety and fear, the first where there is a definite named cause for the feelings, the second where they are vague and generalised.

ALCOHOL ABUSE

Now that smoking is so out of favour, alcohol is the West's last socially-acceptable drug. Because it is so widely available it is easy to forget that it is a powerful poison which can have serious long-term mental and physical effects. Drinking can kill you, after many years of abuse or suddenly and dramatically after a heavy binge. Despite this the simple fact that so many people drink makes it easy for people to deny that they need help even when it is obvious to everyone else that they really do have a problem. What then are the danger signs? See how many of these statements apply to you:

- I find it difficult to have an alcohol-free day.
- I often drink during the day.
- I suffer black-outs so that I don't remember how I got home after a night's drinking.
- I usually drink more than 28 units of alcohol a week (this is equivalent to 14 pints of ordinary-strength beer or 28 glasses of wine; the limit for women is less than this).
- I drink to forget problems or relieve stress.
- I can't go to a party or a restaurant without drinking.
- I have tried in the past to cut down my drinking but I am drinking as much as ever.
- One or both of my parents had a drink problem.
- I often drink alone.
- I seem to drink more and/or faster than my friends.

If you agree with more than a couple of these statements you could have a drink problem. What should you do about it?

The short answer is, stop drinking. But as with any other addiction this can be much easier said than done. Firstly, because alcohol quickly becomes associated in our minds with certain situations and events, such as leaving work in the evening or watching television or coping with social contacts. These emotional triggers lead us to drink regularly and as a matter of course and it can be difficult to avoid them or substitute some other activity when the trigger is pulled. A second reason is that drink provides a short-lived high that makes us feel better about ourselves and makes problems appear less real. The fact that alcohol is a depressant and eventually makes things much worse is often forgotten until it is too late. Finally physical dependency can come, when the body is so used to a daily ration of alcohol that it finds it hard to cope when it is withdrawn. This leads to the symptoms suffered by the confirmed alcoholic: mental impairment, the shakes, hallucinations, sickness and the craving for more drink.

Given that many of the reasons for drinking are emotional or psychological, the Bach Flower Remedies can be a real help, at least in the early stages when a drinking problem is still developing. For example, the following remedies might be useful in particular cases:

- Chestnut Bud for the man who repeatedly tries and fails to stop drinking, or for the man whose drinking is always triggered by the same events.
- Vervain for the highly-strung type who uses alcohol as a way of switching off.
- Agrimony for the man who uses alcohol as a way of drowning his problems instead of facing them.
- White Chestnut for the man whose constant worrying is out of control.
- Mimulus for the shy man who finds it difficult to face social occasions without a drink.
- Centaury for the man who drinks not because he wants to but because he is bullied into it by friends.

- Elm for the normally capable man who turns to drink as a last resort when his responsibilities get too much for him.
- Pine for the man who is guilt-ridden about his drinking but nevertheless is unable to stop.
- Scleranthus for the unreliable types who veer from euphoria to gloom and may turn to drink at either extreme.
- Gentian for the man discouraged from trying to stop drinking because he has tried and failed in the past.

For those with a serious alcohol problem, particularly known or suspected alcoholics, there is an additional consideration to bear in mind. The stock Bach Flower Remedies you buy in the chemist's or the health food shop are preserved in pure brandy. The amount of alcohol involved in taking them is minute, especially if they are diluted in water in the recommended way, but there may still be psychological reasons not to give an alcoholic even this amount. Anyone with a serious alcohol problem needs help from a qualified doctor, and before giving the remedies in such circumstances you are strongly advised to consult the health professional who is dealing with the case.

As well as taking the remedies there are other strategies that can help you to adapt to a booze-free life:

- Take up a new hobby.
- Take the opportunity to get really fit.
- Tell everyone you have stopped drinking – and be proud of your self-control and strength of will.
- Learn how to relax.
- Avoid thinking back to the glories of your drinking days – they are illusory. (Honeysuckle is the remedy to counteract harmful nostalgia.)
- Don't allow yourself to fall into self-pity. (Willow is the remedy for this.)

Finally, if you are having real problems giving up and haven't yet gone to your doctor, do so now. If she (or he) can't help herself she will be able to refer you to people who can. You can also try

Alcoholics Anonymous, who have been helping people who just can't give up for half a century. You will find their number in your local phone book.

CANCER

A cancer is an abnormal growth made up of diseased cells. Many such growths are benign and will not do any great damage. Some, however, are malignant and can affect surrounding healthy cells. Others may be growing somewhere like the brain where the simple fact of their presence will cause a problem. Beyond the physical damage that cancer does there is a deep psychological damage too: the "C" word is one that, for most people, is full of terror.

First, some facts. It is simply not true that cancer is always or nearly always fatal. In fact if treatment starts early enough the prognosis is very good. The treatment itself may involve surgery, radiation therapy, chemotherapy or a combination of all three, depending on the site of the cancer and whether or not it has spread to other areas of the body.

If you are a man in your early thirties the cancer you are most likely to suffer from is cancer of the testes. Fortunately it is curable as long as it is detected in time. For this reason it is a very good idea to learn how to perform a simple self-examination from time to time so that you can consult a doctor as soon as you notice anything out of the ordinary. Here is a step-by-step guide:

1. Cup your right hand under your right scrotum (the bag that contains your testicles)
2. Gently roll your thumb around until it is on top of the egg-shaped ball inside your scrotum (this is your right testicle), keeping your index and middle fingers at the bottom
3. Roll the testicle forwards and back, then from side to side – the testicle should feel firm and smooth, with a knobbly projection on top (the epididymis)
4. Using the left hand, repeat the process for the other testicle

At first this will seem a strange thing to do and you will not really be sure what you are looking for, but after a time you will get to know what is normally there and so be able to tell if there is anything abnormal. If you do find an unexpected lump on your testes don't panic because the vast majority will have nothing to do with cancer. Nevertheless, the best advice is to see your doctor for an expert opinion. You may also encounter an unexpected swelling elsewhere in the scrotum, and again the best advice is to see your doctor. You may have found the beginning of a hernia, a cyst or some other condition that needs treating.

Cancer of the prostate is also a male-only cancer – this is dealt with later on in this chapter. And men who work outside have their own particular cancer risk: skin cancer. In its most dangerous form, malignant melanoma, this has been increasing recently, perhaps as a result of damage to the ozone layer allowing more of the sun's harmful rays to reach the surface of the planet. All the more reason then to follow every doctor's advice and cover up in the heat, use sun creams and sun-blockers, and avoid exposure to the midday sun. Yet still a large proportion of men seem to think that by virtue of being men they are immune to the effects of the sun's radiation. The painful sight of raw red skin is a common one in midsummer. It takes a particular type of courage to start applying sun cream when all around you your mates are sitting in the sun and baking 'like men'. Walnut is the remedy to help overcome the hurdle of contrary circumstances.

There are other cancers which are associated with avoidable risks. Smoking is well-known as the principal cause of lung cancer, as is graphically shown by the fact that as they are drawn to the doubtful pleasures of tobacco in larger numbers so women are catching up with men in the lung cancer league as well. It is perhaps less well known that cancers of the throat, lip and tongue can also be traced to tobacco, so exchanging one form of tobacco for another is no answer. After the craze for chewing tobacco a few years ago people starting turning up at clinics with cancer of the mouth.

There is of course no question of the Bach Flower Remedies directly attacking cancer on a physical level. They simply do not work like that. They are directed against disharmonies in the personality and emotional responses of individuals, not against particular illnesses. But there are two important ways in which they may help. First, they can flood out those negative aspects of the personality and other long-term imbalances that may be the root causes of the disease. Once this is done the body's natural healing mechanism can come back into play and the patient may literally heal himself. The main key to this aspect of the remedies' action is to select the person's type remedy. The second way in which the Bach Flower Remedies can help is to deal with the negative emotions that the diagnosis – even the mention – of cancer often provokes. This makes it easier for the patient to concentrate his energies in a positive way on staying healthy and again may help his body to fight the disease more effectively. Remedies to help achieve this second aim include:

- Rock Rose for terror.
- Star of Bethlehem for shock, either when you hear the diagnosis or even long after, if you have failed to come to terms with it.
- Honeysuckle for useless regrets about past actions that might have contributed to the present problem.
- Oak for the strong man whose search for a cure is relentless but who may drive himself on beyond the limit of his strength.
- Olive for physical tiredness after a long course of treatment, after surgery or during convalescence.
- Willow for resentment and self-pity.
- Wild Rose for apathy which might prevent you taking positive steps to get well.
- Gorse for feelings of despair and hopelessness, when it may seem to you that it is useless to try further treatment.
- Sweet Chestnut for final, black despair and anguish if all possible cures have been tried and have failed.

It is important to stress again that with cancer early diagnosis is often the key to successful treatment. If you think you may be at risk you should see your doctor at once for a proper examination.

CIRCUMCISION

Circumcision is the surgical removal of the foreskin. This is usually done for one of two reasons. As a ritual it has been performed in many cultures, including those of the ancient Egyptians in about 2,300 BC, the Aztecs, the Australian aborigines, the Muslims and of course the Jews. For many peoples it was a sign that the circumcised male had become a man. For others it was a sign that the person undergoing it had accepted the religion and way of life of his people.

The second reason to perform a circumcision is when there is a medical condition that makes it advisable to do so. For example, some men find it difficult to draw their foreskins back so as to uncover the tip of the penis (the glans). This makes it difficult to keep the penis clean properly, which can in turn lead to infection and other health problems. An additional problem when the foreskin is very tight is that the man may experience pain when he has an erection. To resolve these problems, and on the advice of a doctor, a circumcision may be a possible solution.

Circumcision is a relatively minor operation for very young children – Jewish Levitical law, for example, demands that it be done on the eighth day after birth – but even then there can be some adverse emotional reactions. Rescue Remedy is especially recommended as it contains Star of Bethlehem for shock, Rock Rose for terror and Clematis for any feelings of faintness.

The same recommendations will apply to the adult man who has to undergo circumcision. In his case, however, other remedies might be a help before and after the operation. Mimulus is the remedy to deal with anxiety in the days leading up to the operation, and White Chestnut can help if the thought of the ordeal becomes a constant worry. After the operation Crab Apple can help remove any irrational squeamishness at the results of the operation. A loss of confidence in sexual matters may be eased with Larch.

DEPRESSION

Men are far less likely than women to complain of feeling depressed, but this is probably caused by the same conditioning that makes them unlikely to consult doctors generally, in other words the belief that if they are unwell they ought to be able to deal with it themselves. Women do not find it weak or silly to discuss their feelings and so are less likely to bottle up the condition.

The man who can bring himself to seek help will find that there are several Bach Flower Remedies that may be of assistance. For the relatively minor sense of despondency at a setback or an unexpected problem, Gentian is the remedy to select. Where things have got beyond the Gentian state, so that a particular problem has led to feelings of despair and hopelessness, Gorse would be the preferred remedy. Sweet Chestnut is reserved for those people who have tried everything to get themselves out of their predicament but to no avail. People in this state feel that the future is entirely black and that only loneliness and darkness are left. If thoughts turn to suicide Cherry Plum can be added against the uncontrolled violent thoughts. Professional help should also be sought whenever someone is this far into crisis.

All of these states usually come about for a reason. Part of the help offered by a good Bach practitioner is to provide a fresh perspective on the individual's situation so as to suggest ways of improving things. There is another form of depression however, where the person cannot account for his feelings. He may even tick off all the good things in his life and yet still feel a deep and descending gloom. For this motiveless state Mustard is the remedy to choose.

In the psychiatric world there is a distinction made between 'minor' and 'major' depression. Even the Sweet Chestnut state would usually be classed as a minor depression. Minor depressions, although they may be serious while they last, are generally of shorter duration and are comparatively easy to control and reverse. Major depression is, thankfully, much rarer, but it is also a more dangerous condition. It is a full-scale mental illness.

Like minor depression, major depression may be associated with a particular event or be of the Mustard type, unaccountable and seeming to come out of a clear blue sky. The man suffering from major depression may suffer very strong and powerful negative feelings, including guilt, hopelessness and despair. He may exhibit other particular symptoms of mental disorder such as compulsive behaviour, delusions, inability to concentrate, loss of emotional control, insomnia and extreme tiredness. He may lose all interest in looking after himself, leading to malnutrition, weight loss and dehydration. Some people sublimate the depression into an exaggerated fear of disease or death.

These are serious and frightening symptoms, and in addition to these, there is the risk of suicide or, on rare occasions, of violent outbursts against others. When you also take into account the fact that there are numerous, sometimes very dangerous, physical problems that can cause these symptoms, it is clear that trained professional help is called for. The sufferer may need hospitalisation and a great deal of specialist care in order to save him from himself. Where there is major depression the Bach Flower Remedies should only be used in conjunction with the other treatments, and unless you are a fully qualified and accredited doctor or psychiatrist you should never attempt to treat such cases on your own.

You have probably already thought of the remedies that could be given for the different mental states listed above. If not, or if you want to check your selections, here are my suggestions:

- Pine for guilt.
- Gorse for hopelessness.
- Sweet Chestnut for extreme mental anguish.
- Mustard for black gloom that descends for no reason.
- Crab Apple for compulsive behaviour.
- White Chestnut for unwanted, persistent thoughts and for the insomnia and lack of concentration they can cause.
- Heather for hypochondria and tearfulness due to self-obsession.
- Cherry Plum for loss of emotional self-control, and for suicidal or violent outbursts.
- Aspen for unreasonable fear.
- Rock Rose for terror.
- Clematis for inattention due to flights of fancy.
- Olive and Hornbeam for physical and mental weariness respectively.
- Wild Rose for apathy and fatigue.

In practice, it would not be necessary to give all these remedies at the same time, even if all the symptoms were present at once, which is very rare. Selections can almost invariably be narrowed down to six remedies or less. By doing so, the ones chosen will have a better chance of working in a straightforward way.

DRUG ADDICTION

The overwhelming majority of people regularly involved in illicit drug-taking are men. Once again, the reasons appear to lie in the male's increased desire to take risks and to be seen to do so. Drug abuse may also be encouraged by the masculine taboo against dissipating emotions in more healthy ways. In any case, there are reckoned to be three male drug addicts for every female.

Being addicted to drugs is not the same as simply using drugs. You can take sleeping pills for a few weeks and not be addicted to them, just as you can smoke cannabis for a while and then stop without any problem beyond the obvious damage to your lungs that inhaling smoke of any kind may do. For there to be true addiction and real danger to health you have to be a long-term user of drugs and/or unable to stop taking them when you want.

Why do people use drugs? From one perspective the cause is simple. Consumption of any mind-altering substance implies that there is something in his mind that the consumer wants altered. Some people have problems that they are unable to face without some kind of prop. Others are simply curious to know what effect this or that drug will have on them. Some people are in real pain and want it eased and others just want to feel calm and relaxed. But none of these reasons for taking drugs explain why people get addicted to their props.

There are many theories about drug addiction. Some people claim it is simply the end of a long process of cause and effect with its roots in the first taste of cannabis. This is the picture that government anti-drugs campaigns often try to project; but it is rejected by most people with real experience of the area as too simplistic. Others point to the pleasures of particular drugs and the way they are often linked in to a particular lifestyle. There is a lot to this way of thinking, since it shows how buying into a particular type of music or way of dressing often includes the use of certain drugs. The current craze for the drug ecstasy is an obvious example as it is linked to a whole culture of night-clubbing and dance. Those not involved in this culture are unlikely to use it. What this theory fails to explain is why, out of a group of people all involved in the same lifestyle, some will become addicted to drugs while others take or leave them at will.

The explanation for this may lie in the idea of the 'addictive personality' – in other words the belief that the attractions or powers of this or that drug are not as important as the characteristics of the people who take them. Put simply, some people are more likely than others to become addicted to something. The something in question may be alcohol or tobacco or prescribed drugs or illegal 'street' drugs. Often it will be several or all of the above.

You might think that there is a parallel between this theory and Dr Bach's concept of a number of different character types. But it is important not to draw from this apparent similarity the conclusion that addictive personalities are always Centaury or Scleranthus people (for example) or any other of the Bach types. In fact someone is said to have an addictive personality when he feels unhappy with who he is and so seeks an improved version of himself by taking drugs. The reason for the unhappiness might be that he dislikes his appearance (Crab Apple) or suffers from hidden mental torment that other people know nothing about (Agrimony); but it could just as well be that he wants to escape from his own strict nature (Rock Water) or wants to withdraw from present problems by taking refuge in fantasies of future happiness (Clematis). As this suggests, the true parallel between the concept of addictive personalities and the Bach remedies is found in Dr Bach's idea of negative personality aspects and negative mental and emotional states. Since all of the Bach types have their negative sides any of them may in the right circumstances develop addictive personalities.

Perhaps the first thing to do when helping someone with a drug problem is to identify the unhappiness that led him to take drugs in the first place. This will often be linked in some way to his type remedy, so once you have found the one you will often be well on your way to uncovering the second. For example, someone using drugs to cover his painful shyness and give him confidence and self-belief is likely to be a Mimulus person. Although identifying the causes of unhappiness sounds a simple enough thing to do, with drug addicts in particular it can be a difficult job. Firstly, because they are notorious liars. And secondly, because one of the effects of long-term drug use is in fact to change the personality. A suspicious, antagonistic individual in his normal state might be a quiet Centaury type; the apathetic, shoulder-shrugging person could be a dynamic Vervain at heart. Be prepared for a long haul then: addicts are very difficult people to help.

As we have seen, any of the type remedies might be needed. It may be helpful though to have a list of the helper remedies that might be most useful when treating drug addiction, and these would include the following:

- Gentian to overcome setbacks, especially where the person has taken the drug again after a drug-free period and because of this feels he has lost the war. The Gentian is given to remind him that he has only lost a single battle and to give him courage to resume the campaign.
- Walnut for protection against outside influences, one of the trickiest of which will be the opinions and practices of friends who are still involved in the drug world.
- Aspen for vague, uncanny feelings of fear and anxiety. Recovering addicts are particularly inclined to get these fears, which seem to float in the air and have no definite focus.
- Mustard for unaccountable and unpredictable depression and gloom – as with the Aspen fears, Mustard states are relatively common.
- Chestnut Bud for the person who goes back to drugs after every recovery, determined that this time he will remain in control. He never does of course, and the Chestnut Bud remedy is given to help him learn from his past mistakes.
- Crab Apple for negative feelings of shame at one's mental or physical condition.
- Wild Rose for apathy and any tendency to slide back into former habits through lack of will-power.

- Star of Bethlehem for the shock that can come when drugs are suddenly withdrawn.
- White Chestnut to counteract unwanted thoughts about drugs that make it impossible to think positively about other areas of life.

People only start taking drugs because they feel better with them than without them. This means that when they stop taking them they will probably feel worse. The original problems will come flooding back, usually all the stronger for having been repressed. This means that physical withdrawal is only part of the process of cure. The addict also needs to get to know the positive side of his personality, and how to deal with the negative aspects that drove him to drugs in the first place. The Bach Flower Remedies provide both these things in a natural and non-toxic form, but the complex nature of drug dependency means that they will be most effective if they are used in conjunction with other approaches. As a first step, there are numerous agencies that can provide help, advice and treatment if you or someone you know is trying to get off drugs. These include the local social services department, Narcotics Anonymous and Release. You will find the addresses in the phone book. Your family doctor is also a good first port of call as she will be aware what help is on offer and how to go about getting it.

DYSLEXIA

Compared to girls, boys are notoriously slow starters when it comes to learning how to read and write. They are also up to six times more likely than their sisters to be diagnosed as dyslexic, which means that they experience difficulty with reading despite being of normal intelligence and despite having had all the usual encouragement and tuition.

Dyslexia is a term that covers a number of problems. These may have different causes, but most cases seem to be due to a difficulty in breaking up words – spoken or written – into smaller units of sound, known in the jargon as phonemes. Dyslexia is thought to affect between 1 and 10 per cent of the population. If these figures seem surprisingly imprecise, this only reflects the fact that, even today, many dyslexics can reach the end of their education without having had the problem correctly diagnosed. Dyslexia sometimes runs in families so it is, at least in part, an inherited condition. The root of the problem is thought to lie in the brain, which for some unknown reason has developed without the normal biological language abilities. There are other studies, however, which point to the possible influence of environmental factors.

Just as there is no single definite cause so there is no one successful treatment that can be given in every case. Normally, people who have been diagnosed as dyslexic are given extra help of one kind or another. Special books may be provided which are designed to encourage the dyslexic child by leading him into reading gently. Pictures and diagrams might be used to help enhance his understanding of what he is reading. Above all the interested and committed involvement of adults is essential: if this is present there is a good chance that significant progress will be made, and the many famous people who have had to deal with reading problems show that this problem need be no bar to a successful and fulfilled life. Dyslexic people are often of above-average intelligence and can have special gifts in other areas, as if to make up for this one disadvantage.

The Bach Flower Remedies can help people who are trying to overcome their dyslexia. Specific remedies that might be helpful when negative feelings arise include:

- Gentian for discouragement.
- Willow for self-pity and resentment.
- Holly for hatred or envy of a schoolmate or sibling who is doing better.
- Impatiens for frustration at slow progress.
- Larch for lack of confidence.
- Wild Rose for resignation and surrender to circumstances.
- Oak for those who doggedly try again and again and so occasionally feel close to collapse.

For the parents of a dyslexic child, Red Chestnut might help when fears for the child's future are exaggerated so that they do more harm than good. Honeysuckle might be a help to parents who are inclined to regret missed opportunities in the past instead of making new opportunities for themselves and their child in the present.

HAEMOPHILIA

Haemophilia is the name given to an inherited disease in which certain proteins are missing from the blood. As the missing proteins are involved in the clotting of blood, even a minor injury can cause severe and prolonged bleeding. Because of this, haemophiliacs have to be very careful to avoid injuries, and regular treatment with blood clotting agents is necessary.

Only men suffer from the disease. Women can be carriers but never develop the condition itself or any of its symptoms. Transmission is via the X chromosome, (women have two X chromosomes; men have one X and one Y). When a haemophiliac and a non-carrier female conceive, their son will never get the disease. This is because, to be male, the child must have an XY pattern. The Y chromosome can only come from the father so his X chromosome comes from his healthy mother. The daughters of the same union will always be carriers because their XX chromosome pattern must include the father's infected X chromosome. Where the father is healthy and the mother is a carrier the same simple arithmetic dictates that male children will have a 50 per cent chance of getting the disease and females the same chance of being carriers.

Haemophilia is a potentially life-threatening condition and in the past many sufferers died in childhood. Nowadays improved treatment and therapies means there is an excellent prognosis for the disease itself, and the real scourge of haemophiliacs in recent years has come from elsewhere. In the 1980s there were many cases of the HIV virus being transmitted to haemophiliacs in blood products used to treat their condition. Although screening and other procedures are now carried out to ensure that this doesn't happen in the future, this can be of little comfort to those people who have found that their treatment has made their lives worse rather than better.

Particular emotional problems suffered by people with haemophilia could include:

- Named fears, such as the fear of injury, or of passing the disease on to future generations: Mimulus.
- Fear of the effects of the disease on loved ones: Red Chestnut.
- Dislike of the disease and feelings of uncleanness; also squeamishness at the treatment required: Crab Apple.

HAIR LOSS

Hair loss can happen in several ways. The first is the gradual thinning that comes with age, with definite bald spots appearing, and the hairline receding. This is more common and more pronounced in men than in women.

A more dramatic cause of hair loss is the disease of the scalp called *alopecia areata*. This can cause the sufferer to lose most or all of his hair quite literally overnight, although more often the process takes days or weeks to complete. According to some studies this condition may affect as many as one person in a hundred, although the most extreme form of the condition, in which body hair, eyebrows and eyelashes are also lost, is thankfully much rarer.

Hair loss can also be hereditary, or caused by treatments given to correct other diseases: chemotherapy given to fight cancer is the most well-known example.

Just as there are different types of hair loss, so the prognosis for them is different. For the typical balding associated with age, hair transplants can be undertaken. But this is an expensive and potentially dangerous course which should never be undertaken without qualified (and reputable) medical advice. Above all it is wise to avoid the various bogus clinics and miracle cures that advertise their services in the press. They are at best ineffective and at worst extremely dangerous.

Alopecia areata is something of a mystery to medical science, and the hair can start to grow back as quickly and as mysteriously as it once fell out. There are drugs available that may help, but there is no cast-iron remedy that will cure the condition and in many cases all that can be done is to suggest ways that the sufferer can learn to live with the problem. There is no sure treatment either for hereditary baldness; but hair loss due to drug therapy usually clears up once the treatment has finished.

The best solution is to learn how to accept yourself for what you are and get the loss of your hair into proportion. You are still the same valuable person you always were. You can still do all the things you could do before. The remedies can help you to see this so that you will not let the simple loss of hair destroy your life. By helping to remove the unnecessary negative thoughts that are so often felt by people losing their hair, they can also reduce the likelihood of stress making the problem worse. Remedies that may help include:

- White Chestnut for people whose worrying thoughts stop them from concentrating on the rest of their lives.
- Agrimony for people who hide their mental torture behind a cheerful manner. These are the people who make jokes about their baldness but lie awake at night anguishing over it.
- Heather for people whose obsession with the condition of their hair has them telling everyone they meet all about it. Loneliness and self-centredness, not hair loss, is the real problem here, and this is what the remedy is for.
- Honeysuckle for those people who take the loss of their hair as a sign that their youth is over, and who then sink into nostalgia and regret.
- Larch for the loss of confidence that is often associated with hair loss.
- Willow for people who resent the fact that they are losing hair while other people older than them keep theirs. This is the remedy to keep things in perspective and counteract the slide into self-pity.
- Crab Apple for those men who dislike their new appearance and so avoid looking at themselves.
- Walnut for people who need help adjusting to change.
- Star of Bethlehem for shock. This remedy is almost always indicated where hair loss has been sudden, and particularly where it has come at an unusually young age. But it can also help older people who can also be shocked when they lose their hair, however natural and expected the event might appear to the rest of the world.

- Gorse for despair.
- Chestnut Bud for those people who are forever trying the latest miracle hair-restorer and seem unable to learn from bitter experience that they do not work.

HEART DISEASE

Heart disease kills more people in the Western world than any other disease, and in the United Kingdom alone more than 250,000 people a year suffer a heart attack. For most of them the cause of the problem is atherosclerosis – in layman's terms the hardening and narrowing of the arteries due to material building up inside them.

Atherosclerosis restricts the flow of blood to the heart, and the effects of this process can vary from mild angina (chest pains) felt only when taking exercise, all the way to potentially fatal heart attacks.

The stereotypical heart disease sufferer is an overweight, middle-aged man working in a high-pressure job, who smokes and drinks and does not take enough exercise. There is some truth in this caricature, but a fair amount of misunderstanding as well. It is true that men are more likely than women to die from coronary heart disease, although after the menopause women begin to catch up. But middle age is not especially dangerous since risk goes on increasing with age. Stress at work is a factor, but because different things cause stress to different types of people at different times, it is difficult to generalise about what to avoid or who is most at risk. Heart disease is more common among people who work at repetitive, boring jobs than among high-powered company directors, so it may be that too much routine is more stressful than too little. (See Chapter 4 for more on stress.) Excessive weight contributes to the problem, as does lack of exercise, but most doctors would agree that smoking and diet are the two most important factors. The perfect recipe for trouble is a diet high in saturated fats from red meat, cheese and cream, plus the smoking habit.

Obviously your best chance of avoiding heart disease lies in adopting a better lifestyle. Giving up smoking and taking regular exercise should be coupled with a healthier diet: more vegetables, fruit, fish, olive oil, pasta and white meat; less alcohol, animal fats, cakes and chocolate. You should also try to lose weight if you are obese. You don't need to follow a fad diet or starve yourself: just replace the fat and sugar in your diet with fresh fruit and vegetables and do a little exercise. This should help you to lose weight slowly and without any ill effects. If you are having problems with this, your doctor should be able to give you further advice.

If cutting down your heart disease risk factor represents a major change in your way of life you might need some help – and fortunately the remedies are there to provide it. For example:

- Gentian is for the discouragement you might feel when there is a setback.
- Chestnut Bud is for when you repeat the same mistakes over and over again, such as going to a smoky pub after work when you know that you will always end up buying a packet of cigarettes.
- Centaury is for the times you find it hard to say no to people who are trying to get you to do something you know is bad for you.
- Walnut is for protection from habits and other circumstances that stand in the way of your making a successful change.
- Rock Water is for any tendency to go too far with self-denial and become a martyr to your own health.

When other members of their family have suffered in the past from heart disease, some people tend to shrug their shoulders and say that there is nothing they can do since it 'runs in the family'. For this kind of attitude Wild Rose is the remedy. In fact in most cases the occurrence of heart disease in several members of one family can be put down to their having shared a particular diet or way of living. It has been demonstrated many times that, for example, the children of heavy smokers are more likely to smoke themselves, and as families share meals together parents tend to pass on their eating habits to their children.

As the Wild Rose example suggests, the individual's personality can be the key to more effective prevention. For example, Agrimony people can repress their worries and try to drown problems under good living and drink. Neither the stress they cause themselves nor the alcohol they consume will do them any good. And for their different reasons Rock Water and Vervain people can work too hard and fail to rest and relax even when they are advised to do so by a doctor. In these and other cases, finding your type remedy can be a major step to avoiding health problems generally and heart problems in particular. Nevertheless even if you do manage to make the required changes to your lifestyle and iron out negative attitudes, you will not have removed entirely all possibility of your suffering from heart disease. Some men will always suffer from heart disease – being a man is one of the risk factors, after all – so it is as well to know a little about what can happen.

Heart attacks are probably the best known manifestation of heart disease, but in fact angina is far more common. Angina causes pain or discomfort in the chest, jaw or arms, and usually comes when the person is engaged in some activity such as exercising, digging the garden or making love. It is also known for strong emotions such as anger to provoke an attack, and undue excitement can also take its toll. Once the activity that provoked the attack ceases the pain passes after a short time. The seriousness of an angina attack depends on how badly the arteries are affected, but in most cases there is an excellent prognosis and with the help of drugs and appropriate lifestyle changes (including gentle and sensible exercise) the condition can be managed with great success.

Heart attacks are more dramatic and generally more immediately dangerous. A heart attack is a fast-developing problem in an artery which is already diseased, and is caused by a clot forming and blocking the artery either completely or in part. The patient suffers intense pain in his chest and may feel breathless and nauseous. The pain may spread to his arms and jaw and lasts for twenty or more minutes. The part of the heart supplied by that artery dies away. If the affected area is small then the person has suffered a minor attack and will in all likelihood make a full recovery. If a large enough area of the heart muscle is damaged then the attack can be fatal. Between 5 and 10 per cent of people arriving at hospital after suffering a heart attack die from it.

Even a relatively mild heart attack can be accompanied by great anxiety, even panic, both in the person experiencing the attack and in those around him. Rescue Remedy is useful for helping keep people calm while they are waiting for the ambulance to arrive. Rock Rose for terror is the main remedy being called on at such times. Following the attack, it is normal for the recovering patient to feel depressed and vulnerable at this dramatic sign of his mortality. Gentian can be given at this stage to help counteract despondency. Guilt can also be a problem if the victim feels he has brought trouble on himself and on his family by his actions or inaction. Pine is the remedy to turn this negative emotion to positive account.

It cannot be stressed enough that heart disease is a potentially fatal physical disease and that anyone who thinks he might be suffering from it should see a qualified medical practitioner for a diagnosis. There are various treatments available, ranging from drugs that can reduce stress on the heart, impede clotting and lower the amount of fat in the blood, all the way up to coronary bypass operations which replace damaged sections of artery, and as a last resort full-scale heart transplants. The Bach Flower Remedies can be used alongside these therapies to help counteract the mental and emotional effects of the condition, such as fear and depression. This can be a vital part of treatment.

For example, depression is often a particular problem for people who have had to undergo an operation to correct a heart problem (or indeed any other kind of operation). This might seem strange, as the period following a successful treatment should be a happy one, and in fact most people describe their depression as unreasonable. Mustard is the remedy to give for this kind of black, motiveless gloom, which will usually last for a few days only. For a groundless, vague fear of the future, Aspen can be given. Other remedies might be more appropriate in some cases. For example, any fear that loved ones will not be able to cope would be treated with Red Chestnut, while specific fears, such as being afraid to take exercise in case it brings the angina back, would be treated with Mimulus. Heart disease is widely (and wrongly) thought to be more often fatal than not, and the fear of what might happen can easily heighten stress and so help to bring about the outcome that is most feared.

HEARTBURN

The correct medical term for heartburn is cardialgia – but however unfamiliar this name may be the symptoms are well-known enough: a burning sensation in the stomach or under the breastbone, sometimes accompanied by a sour taste in the throat. Heartburn is caused by a weakness in the lower sphincter, a muscle that controls the opening from the oesophagus (the tube that food goes down when you swallow) into the stomach. Normally the lower sphincter only opens very briefly to allow food into the stomach, but in some cases it doesn't shut fast enough and allows acid to wash back into the oesophagus. It is this that causes the burning sensation. When you are lying down more acid is likely to wash back. This explains why people commonly become aware of an attack when they are going to bed.

There are any number of factors that are known to cause the sphincter to stop working efficiently. Stress is one. Drinking alcohol, tea and coffee are others, as are smoking and over-eating. Normally the symptoms do not last long and there is no need to seek medical treatment. Drinking a little water or taking a medicine designed to counteract acid in the stomach is usually enough (these preparations are known collectively as antacids). In some cases the problem can be more severe or occur so often that the person's everyday life is interrupted. This may require medical treatment, usually with larger doses of antacids. Depending on the person's medical history, age and lifestyle there may be further investigations to rule out heart disease and ulcers, both of which may cause similar symptoms. Because of this possibility anyone suffering more than mild symptoms should seek medical advice.

In general, though, a few simple changes in the person's lifestyle are enough to stop heartburn becoming a problem. These include:

- Finding ways to avoid and deal with stress.
- Avoiding alcohol and drinks containing caffeine.
- Cutting down smoking.
- Not eating for three hours before going to bed.

Where stress is felt to be a factor in causing heartburn then there are a number of Bach Flower Remedies that might help. For people who put themselves under pressure because they are always in too much of a hurry, Impatiens is the remedy to choose. Impatiens people are likely to eat too fast as well, which can also lead to heartburn and indigestion generally. Where overwork leads to stress, Oak is the remedy for the relentless plodder, Elm for the man whose sense of responsibility for others leads him into trouble, and Vervain for the vivacious enthusiast who finds it hard to switch off.

If you find it hard to cut down on tea, coffee, alcohol or cigarettes there are other remedies that you might consider. If any of these steps represents a major change in your lifestyle, Walnut might be a help. Chestnut Bud is for people who repeat the same ill-considered actions again and again, so this too could be a good remedy to select. If you find yourself getting irritable and short-tempered with people you could try Impatiens or Beech, depending on whether your feelings are caused more by lack of patience or by intolerance of other people's behaviour.

HERNIA

A hernia is caused when part of an internal organ protrudes through the tissue which contains it. The commonest type of hernia is an inguinal hernia, which occurs in the groin (the word inguinal is from the Latin for groin). This affects men more often than women, and for two main reasons. First, the spermatic cord goes through the wall of the abdomen near the groin area and provides a natural weak spot. Second, hernias are especially associated with heavy lifting, and in general such jobs are more likely to be done by men.

There are many other types of hernia, all named after the part of the body that protrudes or the area in which the hernia occurs. Some, like the diaphragmatic hernia, which occurs when the intestines protrude up through the diaphragm, are entirely internal and can be very painful, requiring surgical intervention in some cases. Hernias in the groin area do not usually hurt, and in most cases are simply supported with a truss which gently pushes the protrusion back into place. Physical exertion should be avoided as any sudden strain may make the condition worse.

Hernias are an entirely physical phenomenon and the best treatment for them is that described above. A possible role for the

Bach Flower Remedies is to help overcome any emotional responses or character traits that might get in the way of recovery. For example some men seem unable to rest and avoid strenuous exercise despite instructions from doctors, and there are various remedies that might be helpful. Rock Water is for people who expect too much of themselves and refuse to deviate from their normal routine. Oak is for the strong, steady man who grinds on as before even when he knows he ought to stop. Vervain is for the enthusiast, so fired up by the needs of the moment that he neglects the importance of pacing himself. Impatiens is for the man who becomes irritable at the least frustration and may rush back to his former habits too soon. Then there are the authoritarians who always assume they know better than anyone else and refuse to take advice from anyone. Vine is the remedy to help them listen so that they can grow in wisdom.

Other men may feel squeamish at the thought of a hernia, especially an external one. Crab Apple is the remedy to cleanse such feelings. Lack of confidence may be a problem after recovery is complete, so that the person is hesitant about resuming a physically demanding job even when he is assured it is safe to do so. Larch may be a help in such cases.

HIGH BLOOD PRESSURE

Blood pressure is commonly expressed in two figures, like this: 120/80, 150/90 and so on. The first figure in each case is the blood pressure when the heart is contracting (the systolic pressure). The second lower figure is the pressure when the heart is at rest between beats (the diastolic pressure). Problems can start when either the systolic or diastolic pressures are higher than normal – and the idea of 'normal' itself is subject to revision according to the age of the person and any other medical conditions he might be suffering. Readings as low as 140/90 may be cause for concern in a young man who drinks and smokes to excess, but they would be considered acceptable in a middle-aged man leading a reasonably healthy life.

However it is defined, high blood pressure can go on for years undetected and will not necessarily cause any obvious symptoms. For this reason it is a good idea for men over 35 to have their blood pressure checked at yearly intervals, especially if they are overweight or other members of their families have suffered strokes or heart attacks. The reason for keeping a track on blood pressure is that men in their 40s and 50s with high blood pressure are ten times more likely to go on to suffer a stroke, and there is also a greatly increased risk of heart disease. This is because the high pressure strains and causes damage to the arteries, eventually making the formation of blood clots more likely.

The best way to avoid and treat high blood pressure is to get into shape and live a healthier life. If you are overweight, you need to take steps to get back into the acceptable weight range for your height. For example, if you are 6 feet tall you should weigh between 10 stone 8 pounds and 13 stone 2 pounds: anything over 15 stone 11 is classified as 'obese'. You should also drink no more than three units of alcohol per day (a unit is half a pint of beer, a glass of wine or a measure of spirits) and try to cut down on the amount of salt you take. Regular exercise is a good idea – although if you are suffering from high blood pressure you ought to consult your doctor before you make anything more than the slightest change to the amount of exercise you do. There is also some benefit to be gained by taking steps to reduce the amount of stress in your life. (See Chapter 4 of this book for more on stress.)

If you smoke, stop.

Making these changes in the way you live will inevitably involve some heart-searching and a few hard decisions. The Bach Flower Remedies can be a help when things become difficult, and the indications for their use in this case will be the same as in all others – in other words they should be selected according to the personality and current feelings of the individual concerned. See the sections in this chapter on smoking, diet and exercise for more information.

For most people, living more healthily will be enough to keep blood pressure normal. However there is a substantial minority who will not be helped sufficiently by these measures. These people will probably need medication. Common drugs given include diuretics, whose main action is to increase the amount and frequency of urine passed, and beta-blockers.

INDIGESTION

Indigestion is a term used to cover a number of unpleasant sensations that follow eating and drinking. These include belching, heartburn, nausea, stomach ache, wind and even vomiting. Usually the symptoms quickly fade, but where they are long-lasting or recur frequently there may be some underlying medical condition that needs treatment, such as ulcers or an infection. For this reason severe or chronic indigestion should be referred to a doctor.

For simple indigestion it is important to stick to a good healthy diet and not to drink too much alcohol, tea or coffee. Far from being the aid to digestion that it was once thought to be, smoking is also implicated in many cases so you should try to stop smoking or at least cut down the number of cigarettes you smoke. Emotional distress of any kind can cause temporary indigestion as well, and in these cases the Bach Flower Remedies can of course be used to relieve the causative emotional state and so indirectly help the discomfort. The remedies to select in such cases would depend entirely on the feelings the person was experiencing and on the type of person he was, as for example:

- Impatiens for hasty people who put themselves under stress and do not give themselves time to digest their food properly.
- Chestnut Bud for people who fail to learn from experience and so eat or drink unwisely again and again.

MUSCULAR DYSTROPHY

This is an inherited disease caused by a faulty gene. The symptoms are a gradual wasting away of the muscles, resulting in loss of strength and eventually loss of the ability to walk so that patients usually end up confined to a wheelchair.

There are several forms of the disease which affect men and women equally, but one type is confined almost exclusively to men. This is Duchenne muscular dystrophy, named after the 19th century French neurologist who first described it, and it is one of the most severe forms of the disease. It usually starts in the early years of childhood with the pelvic and trunk muscles the first to be affected. This leads early on to deformation of the spine and difficulty with walking. By adulthood all the muscles may have been affected and the prognosis is not good, with death often resulting from respiratory or heart failure. People suffering from other forms of the disease may, however, live to an advanced age and the progress of the disease may be much slower. There is no specific cure for any form of muscular dystrophy, including Duchenne's, so orthodox treatment is largely confined to physiotherapy.

As this is such a serious disease it would be foolish and wrong to hold out hope of a miracle cure. Nevertheless there is little doubt that a person's mental and emotional state do have an effect on the progression of illnesses of all sorts. Even when there is no hope of cure, sufferers can be helped to find peace in themselves and gain joy and hope from their lives. With this in mind, the following remedies might be among the first to consider when things go wrong:

- Gorse for hopelessness and despair at the idea that nothing more can be done.
- Hornbeam for mental weariness at the thought of the day to come.
- Mimulus for fear of the illness and of its consequences.
- Red Chestnut for the altruistic fear of what the disease might mean to loved ones.
- Oak for the positive person who will try anything to be well and overcome disabilities, but who occasionally feels tired and on the point of surrender when the effort becomes too much.
- Sweet Chestnut for the extreme mental torture experienced when there seems no light or hope left in the world.
- Wild Rose for apathetic resignation and surrender to the illness.
- Crab Apple for shame felt at one's physical condition.

PROSTATE TROUBLE

The prostate gland is one of the glands that is used to produce semen. It is wrapped around the tube that leads from the bladder to the penis. As men grow older, so the prostate gland can enlarge, and when it does so the tube carrying urine is gradually closed off. This leads to the familiar symptoms of prostate trouble: reduced flow of urine, the inability to drain the bladder completely, and the need to urinate very frequently – eight or more times during the day, or a couple of times at night. Other symptoms may include incontinence, pain when urinating and retention. Of course, any or all of these symptoms may be caused by a number of other conditions as well, some of them serious, so if you are experiencing them you should consult your qualified medical practitioner as a matter of course.

The risk of prostate enlargement increases markedly with age. At 35, only about 2 per cent of men will have their prostates enlarged enough to cause symptoms; at 75, the figure will be nearer to 20 per cent. Most of the time the enlargement will be benign, in other words not in itself dangerous. But in a small proportion of men the prostate can be malignant, which means that it is cancerous and must be treated. This is another good reason to see the doctor at once if you suspect you might have an enlarged prostate. However, it is important to stress that there is no link between benign prostate enlargement and cancer: you will not develop cancer because you have a benign enlargement.

If when you go to the doctor you are found to be suffering from an enlarged prostate gland there are a number of possible next steps. The doctor may decide not to intervene but to continue monitoring the situation. If the problem is not affecting the quality of your life, this can be the best policy since it avoids unnecessary treatment. There is no reason to assume that the symptoms will get worse since the amount of obstruction may remain constant even if the gland continues to swell. In some cases drugs can be given to reduce the obstruction. If the problem is severe, surgery might be recommended to remove the enlarged gland.

The Bach Flower Remedies cannot in themselves cure your prostate trouble, of course, since they do not act on the physical level. However they can help you to deal with the mental and emotional states that accompany the problem and help you take a more positive view of your situation. By achieving a more balanced frame of mind and becoming more relaxed about things you may well find that the more troublesome symptoms of prostate enlargement are themselves eased.

The key as always is to look at your own individual personality and emotional state. For example:

- If you feel despondent about your condition choose Gentian.
- If you are very pessimistic and convinced that nothing will be able to help you choose Gorse.
- If you are feel frustrated and irritated by your need to keep going to the toilet choose Impatiens.
- If you feel sorry for yourself and perhaps bitter that you should be the victim of this problem while other men remain unaffected choose Willow.
- If you are frightened that everyone notices how often you go to toilet and this makes you shy and self-conscious choose Mimulus.
- If you are annoyed at your loss of self-control and are determined to regain mastery choose Rock Water.
- If you are disgusted at what has happened to your body choose Crab Apple.

SMOKING

The message on smoking is simple: don't. Unlike alcohol, there is no such thing as a sensible level of smoking. Even a single cigarette a day can cause lung cancer and the substitutes for cigarettes are hardly less noxious, with the potential to cause lip and throat cancer and respiratory problems. The dangers spread out to other people too. The children of smokers are not only more likely to take up the habit themselves, they are also more likely to suffer from ear, nose and throat infections and bronchitis. Some studies have indicated that growth rate and intelligence will also be impaired. People forced to inhale other people's smoke are twice as likely to develop lung cancer; the risk of heart disease is also doubled.

In fact most smokers are well aware of these facts. Every study done shows that the vast majority of smokers want to join the millions who have already given up. If they don't do so it is because giving up smoking is a very hard thing to do.

When I gave up smoking in 1991 I was smoking around 30 cigarettes a day. I had been trying to give up for well over a year, and in the end I'm convinced that I only managed it because I was so sickened by my own lack of will power. For months I would find myself thinking back to my smoking days and fantasising about how nice and pleasant they had been. Honeysuckle would have been the remedy to counteract this tendency to nostalgia and living in the past. White Chestnut would have helped calm unwanted, repetitive thoughts about smoking. To stop myself from rushing out to the tobacconists I would imagine that I had just finished smoking a cigarette and think how depressed I would now feel at having abandoned the effort yet again, and of how my life would not in fact be better for having smoked but a whole lot worse. If that didn't work I would think about what the smoke would do to my lungs, and imagine a broken fingernail scratching away on soft tissue, and sheer squeamishness would stop me from going back to tobacco.

These are the techniques that worked for me, but in the end you have to find your own way. Some people find it easier to stop at the same time as a friend. Others take up running, swimming or aerobics so as to reinforce the healthy life they are working towards. Others still prefer to shut themselves away from temptation for a few weeks, avoiding company and spending entire evenings reading or watching television. Some throw away all their cigarettes, ashtrays and matches the night before the attempt while others like to leave an unopened packet of cigarettes in full view as a reminder of what is being achieved. Whatever works for you is right.

If you find that without tobacco you are becoming irritable and impatient with others, you might benefit from some simple relaxation techniques such as deep breathing and muscle relaxation. Impatiens is the remedy Dr Bach recommended for irritable feelings, so this too is worth trying.

Those smokers who, like me, make attempt after attempt to give up only to fall back into their previous habits might benefit from Chestnut Bud. This is the remedy for people who repeat mistakes and fail to learn the lessons of experience. The vague feelings of unease and nervousness that some new non-smokers feel could be helped by Aspen, while any feelings of being out of control without nicotine would call for Cherry Plum.

It is very important when you are trying to stop smoking not to weaken and have one more cigarette for old time's sake. As soon as you do so the craving for tobacco will return, and it is all too easy to say to yourself 'well, it didn't work this time so I might as well try again next month'. Try to be a non-smoker from the word go, then – but if you do weaken try also not to let the loss of a battle lead to the loss of the war. Gentian is the remedy to overcome a setback without letting it spoil the progress you have already made. Centaury strengthens the ability to say 'no'. Crab Apple will cope with feelings of disgust and shame at your failure to be true to yourself, and Pine with useless guilt and self-reproach.

Finally there are those people who are convinced that they will never be able to give up smoking. They use this lack of confidence as an excuse to go on without even trying. For such people Larch is the remedy indicated to give them the confidence to go forward and at least make an attempt at a healthier lifestyle. Wild Rose types are similar to Larch people in that they do not even try – but in their case it is an overriding feeling of apathy that stops them from changing. The remedy in this case is given to give them a sense of purposefulness so that they can see that change is not only possible, but worthwhile and meaningful as well.

SPORTS INJURY

You could argue that being at risk from a sports-related injury is, in a way, a good sign, since it at least shows that you are taking some exercise. But in fact sports injuries would be comparatively rare if more people applied a little basic common sense to their activities. By not doing too much all at once, building up fitness gradually, using the correct equipment, learning the appropriate techniques and wearing the right clothing you can avoid most of the ordinary injuries. The fact that sports injuries are still so common shows how uncommon common sense really is.

There is no room here to describe the many different types of injury that playing a sport can lead to. Broadly speaking they will come either as a result of accident (a fall perhaps, or an over-enthusiastic rugby tackle) or overuse (doing more than your body can cope with). For most minor injuries simple first aid and rest are all that is required. In addition Rescue Remedy can usefully be taken to deal with the affects of shock, pain, faintness or fear that you may feel: four drops in water is the recommended dose, but it can be dropped on the tongue straight from the bottle if necessary. If there is any possibility that there has been more serious damage, such as a broken bone, stress fracture, ligament damage or any injury to the head, neck or spine, then professional medical treatment should always be sought. This is one of those areas where conventional Western medicine really is the best in the world, and you should not hesitate to use it.

Once you have seen your doctor and have been patched up you will almost certainly be told to take things easy for a while rather than going straight back to your favourite sport. This is good advice but not always easy to take, especially if exercise is an important part of your life. But it cannot be stressed enough that returning too soon to your normal level of activity could be very dangerous, leading perhaps to a recurrence of the injury, often in a more severe form.

The same considerations apply where a period of inactivity is caused by an illness. For example, going out for a run when you are still recovering from flu (or when you are just starting to feel its onset) can lead to much more serious illnesses such as myocarditis (inflammation of the heart). Patience is a necessary virtue if you don't want to do yourself long-term damage. On the other hand you may find it difficult to summon up the enthusiasm to get back into training after a long lay-off. Both of these problems are mental and emotional ones: here then is where the remedies can play a role in your recuperation. For example:

- Impatiens can help counteract any impatient desire to rush back too soon to your previous level of activity.
- Hornbeam can help restore your mental energy when a slow recuperation has left you weary and struggling to get yourself going again.
- Cerato can help you trust your own judgement so that you will wait until the right time to go back into training, rather than asking for the advice of friends and acquaintances.
- In a similar vein, Centaury would be the remedy to choose if

the other members of your team are bullying you to get back into training too early and you are having trouble saying no.

- Gentian can help overcome the setback of the injury so that you can take a positive attitude towards getting fit and well again.
- Mimulus can help if you really do want to resume the sport but are frightened of the injury happening again.
- Scleranthus can help if you are unsure whether or not to go back to the sport.
- Walnut can help you take the necessary step forward if it really is time to stop playing this sport either because of injury or because of age, but you are held back from the change by habit or other unwanted influences.

ULCERS

Peptic ulcers happen when the mucus that normally protects the lining of the stomach fails, allowing stomach acid and the enzyme pepsin to attack the lining itself. This is obviously more likely to happen if the contents of the stomach are more acidic than usual, and the fact that caffeine and nicotine can both stimulate the production of acid explains why people at risk of ulcers are well advised to avoid both. Emotions such as anger and irritation have also been implicated in the production of ulcers, along with stress of all kinds. Aspirin is a problem since it too can weaken the protective mucus.

The main symptom of a peptic ulcer is an intense burning pain in the abdomen which goes when you have something to eat. Men are twice as likely as women to suffer from ulcers, and people generally are at more risk the older they get. There is some evidence of an hereditary link, but it remains tenuous.

If they are treated early enough there is no reason to fear ulcers. Dangers arise only when they are allowed to spread to a more vulnerable part of the body. For example, if an ulcer spreads into an artery there may be severe internal bleeding. If it eats its way through the stomach wall in the process known as perforation, it causes the acute and potentially fatal disease peritonitis. And if it spreads to the pancreas it gives rise to the equally dangerous disease pancreatitis.

The usual treatment for a peptic ulcer is to give antacids, chemicals which neutralise the acid in the stomach and so give the ulcer a chance to heal. In addition, sufferers are usually advised to avoid spicy foods, caffeine and nicotine, to eat more fibre, and to eat frequent small meals. The other main part of the treatment is to learn how to deal with emotions and stress more successfully, and it is with this element in particular that the Bach Flower Remedies can be so helpful. The following remedies are among those that might be considered depending on the needs and characteristics of the individual being treated:

- Holly for hatred and bad temper caused by hatred.
- Impatiens for irritation and frustration caused by impatience.
- Beech for irritation caused by intolerance of others.
- Rock Water for self-repression and too hard a drive for personal perfection.
- Mimulus for nervousness and anxiety at known causes.
- Agrimony for mental torture that is not outwardly expressed.
- Cherry Plum for hysteria and loss of control.
- Vine for the need to dominate and control others.
- Pine for all-consuming guilt and self-blame.
- Vervain for tension caused by extreme mental effort.
- White Chestnut for ceaseless worry.
- Water Violet for loneliness and the inability to unbend towards others.
- Willow for festering resentment and bitterness.

Usually peptic ulcers are found in the area of the stomach known as the duodenum. If the ulcer is found further up in the stomach there is a chance that there may be a more serious condition such as stomach cancer involved. Because of this possibility, and the dangers associated with all untreated peptic ulcers, you should always see a qualified medical professional if you think you might be suffering from an ulcer.

WEIGHT CONTROL

When a woman is overweight she tends to put on weight around her buttocks and thighs. Men usually develop a paunch around their middles. From an aesthetic point of view there is little to choose between the two. But looked at from the point of view of health men have the worst of the deal since there is a definite link between paunches and heart disease, whereas heavy backsides do not seem to carry any significant health risk. Being overweight also leaves you more liable to a whole range of other disorders, from gallstones and varicose veins to arthritis and strokes.

Probably the easiest way to see if you are overweight is to pinch yourself just above the navel and see if you can get hold of an inch of fat – or in the words of the old television advertisement try to 'pinch more than an inch'. If you think you might be overweight you can then think about how you should respond.

One thing you should not do is panic. Drastic dieting is actually counter-productive as the body quickly goes into starvation mode, working more efficiently and burning up less energy than before. You may lose weight at first but as soon as you try to return to a normal diet you will put on weight faster than ever before as your body stores up fat instead of burning it. Also, avoid the kind of fashionable diet that is trumpeted in the tabloid newspapers. Like crash diets they may work for a time but in the long run they do not work consistently or well.

What you should do is aim to lose a very small amount of weight, and lose it very slowly. Rather than following an all-or-nothing diet look to make small but lasting changes in the food you eat, substituting fruit for chocolate bars, grilled food for fried and so on. At the same time try to take more exercise. And cut down the amount of alcohol you drink. Not only is alcohol fattening in itself, but it slows down the rate at which you burn energy and can help to weaken your resolve at crucial times.

You also need to become more weight conscious. This doesn't mean that you need to weigh yourself every morning (or every week) or never eat another chip. It just means that you need to notice if you are putting on weight so that you can adjust your diet appropriately. Successful weight control should be as smooth as good driving. A slight adjustment to the steering and a light touch on the brake are all that are needed as long as you can see trouble far enough ahead and take appropriate action. Remedies that might help keep you in the driving seat include:

- Scleranthus if you waste time dithering over whether to diet or not.
- Cerato if you ask everyone else's opinion about your weight but do not trust the one opinion that really matters: yours.
- Chestnut Bud if you repeatedly try to diet and repeatedly fail, usually for the same avoidable reasons.
- Hornbeam if you lack the energy and resolve to start the diet today.
- Gentian if you suffer a setback in your diet and feel inclined to throw in the towel.
- Impatiens if you are tempted into crash diets by your impatience for immediate results.

Finally, those people who go in for comfort eating when they are worried or under stress can use the Bach Flower Remedies as a gentler way of finding respite. The remedy to select will depend on the nature of the feelings concerned: White Chestnut, Mimulus, Elm, Impatiens and Rock Water are just a few of the remedies that might be appropriate in particular cases.

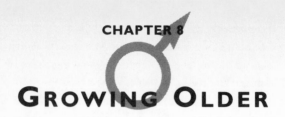

CHAPTER 8

GROWING OLDER

RETIREMENT

Retirement is the end of one of life's longest chapters, but for some it is also the opening of a new chapter, one that promises to be just as exciting as the one they just finished. People who see retirement like this tend to look forward impatiently to the day they will stop work. They are full of plans for new activities, and pop up in newspaper reports about octogenarians gaining PhD's, starting businesses and travelling the world. Their main trouble in retirement is finding enough time to do all the things they want to do.

Other men just coast into retirement, living their lives much as before but with more time for thinking and reading. These are quieter people, but in their own ways their years of rest and reflection are as valuable and as pleasant as those of their more active brothers.

Others are not so sanguine at the prospect. In a world where so many define their worth by what they do – which means in the vast majority of cases, what they do to earn money – the end of their working life comes as a great strain. Far from taking pleasure at the thought of retirement they see it as something to be put off as much as possible. When the day finally comes, as it will for almost everyone who is lucky enough not to die in harness, they don't feel they are opening a new chapter at all. Instead they believe in their hearts that they are closing the book. This is seen in the fact that men over sixty stand less than a fifty-fifty chance of still being alive three years after retiring, and in the statistics that show how the rate of both attempted and successful male suicides also rise at this time. It is hard to avoid the thought that after retirement many men simply lose the will to live.

Depending on when you retire you could easily have 20, 30 or more years of active life in front of you. At the risk of sounding glib, you have everything to live for. You are entering the time that has come to be called the 'third age': the time when you are freed from the need to earn a living and from the responsibility of raising children. It is a time that you should differentiate very clearly from the 'fourth age', which is the (ideally) very short period of illness and decline before death. And just as you would never seriously consider trying to settle into a fixed way of life in the first thirty years of your life, so it is a bad idea to try to dig a permanent rut for yourself in the last thirty. The ideal would be to make your third age as exciting, life-enhancing and enriching as your first age (childhood) or your second (work and child-rearing).

But even the people who look forward to giving up boring and uninspiring jobs may find that being retired is not as much fun as they thought it would be. The loss of a regular structure to the day can be upsetting. The ill-prepared man is easily driven into the comfort zone of television and a daily trip to the shops. Before he knows where he is, the routine of meaningless work has been replaced by a routine of meaningless housework. The days are full and he never has time to carry out his great plans, but nothing is ever achieved and he vegetates quietly towards death, looking forward only to the repetition tomorrow of today's trivia.

The reduction in income on retirement can also bring problems. Unless he is one of the lucky few to receive a large golden handshake and a generous pension, the loss of buying power can make it difficult to make ends meet, let alone finance the rose-covered cottage and foreign holidays he has been dreaming about. Useless regrets that he didn't save more when he was earning will only add to his feelings of frustration and resentment at the way things have worked out.

The answer to all these problems lies in the years leading up to retirement. Successful retirement is like a successful career in that you have to plan before you start. Specifically you need to:

- Decide exactly what you are going to do when you retire.
- Make plans now so that you will be able to do it.

For example, your great dream on retiring might be to complete your education. At the moment all you have is a vague ambition, so the first thing to do is narrow things down a bit so that you know exactly what you are going to do. What subject do you want to study? Do you want a recognised qualification at the end or are you interested in the subject for its own sake? Is there some other ambition lying behind the first one?

Let's say that after asking these questions you decide that you want to get a part-time university degree in historical research and that later on you want to apply your skills to writing a history of your local town. Now you need to start planning the how of your enterprise. Firstly, set aside money while you are working to pay the university fees and buy the books and other materials you will need during and after the course. Then get the prospectuses from your local universities and find which ones offer the course you want. Find out what you have to do to get admitted. Most educational establishments are keen to welcome mature students into their classrooms because of the different perspective and wider experience they can bring to debate, but you might still have to satisfy entrance requirements even if they only amount to an application form and an informal interview. As retirement gets closer, apply for your place so that you know before you leave work when you will start your new life as a student. Finally, have a back-up plan in case things don't work out first time around. The university might cancel a course if there is not enough interest in it, but there might be similar courses elsewhere or other ways of approaching the same subject. Ask for advice and you will get it.

The benefits of arranging your retirement while you are still working are two-fold. In the first place you are putting yourself in control of the situation and giving yourself a reason to look forward to a life beyond the end of work. In the second place you are making it far more likely that your dreams of an ideal retirement will come true. If you find difficulty doing these things, or if you would just like to discuss your prospects and plans with someone else, there are plenty of places to go to for help. There is the Pre-Retirement Association, which is dedicated to helping people prepare to retire. You can get self-study packs from the Open University, and local colleges and Adult Evening Institutes will often run short courses in retirement skills. Not only will these give you lots of valuable information, but they will also give you the chance to meet other people in the same situation you are in, and you may well learn as much from your fellow-students as you do from the instructor. The Citizens' Advice Bureau can point you towards other agencies and sources of information and help.

Probably the first Bach Flower Remedy to consider as retirement approaches is Walnut. This is the link-breaking remedy, and would be especially useful for those who find that their old habits are preventing them from making a successful transition to their new status. The normally capable man who feels overwhelmed at the thought of having to retire, so that he finds it hard to cope with even trivial tasks, is perhaps an Elm type and so would benefit from this remedy when things seem too much. On the other hand the Oak man may simply get on with the daily grind, pushing aside thoughts of retirement so successfully that when the fateful day comes it is almost like a bolt from the blue, and leaves him undone quite suddenly. For a wholly different reason people of the Vine type may experience difficulty adjusting to retirement. Since they are used to being in charge and to telling other people what to do they may try to transfer their habits of command into their home lives. This can make life very difficult for their loved ones and make retirement a burden to all concerned.

Another danger is a decline into triviality. It is all too easy to fill your days with humdrum activity and never do anything really exciting or interesting. Heather people may become like this if they get too wrapped up in their minor problems with health, money and other trivia. Crab Apple men are particularly inclined to enmesh themselves in obsessive, compulsive rituals built up around unimportant activities such as doing the washing up or the daily shopping. Where this effectively prevents them from getting more out of life the remedy can be useful to wash away these petty concerns and give them a truer perspective on themselves and their real desires. Wild Rose people may also get caught up in triviality, although in their case the root cause is apathy rather than compulsive behaviour. Hornbeam would be given instead if the weary feelings were at the thought of an action only and went once an activity was started.

Where fear is felt when approaching or entering the retirement years Mimulus would normally be the remedy to select if the fear could be named. This would apply for example to fear of loneliness, fear of not having enough money and fear of being bored. For those people who are filled with feelings of impending doom as retirement comes, perhaps with an exaggerated and unhelpful fear of disease or even death, Aspen would be more appropriate. And Red Chestnut would be preferred where the fear centred on how loved ones were going to cope with less money coming into the house.

These are some of the remedies that retired people most often need to help them to live their third ages in positive ways, but they are of course not the only ones to consider. Others that might come in useful from time to time would include:

- Honeysuckle for nostalgia and a tendency to let thoughts of the past interfere with enjoyment of the present.
- Willow for resentment and self-pity.
- Clematis where daydreams about the future prevent actions needed now to help make those dreams come true.
- Larch for lack of confidence that prevents someone trying something new.
- Cerato for insecure people who need to have their decisions confirmed by others.
- Holly for envy of younger people who are just starting out on their careers.

GETTING OLDER

In late middle age men can seem luckier than women in that they have on average fewer wrinkles and so appear younger. But the difference is literally skin-deep, and this advantage is soon buried under an avalanche of disadvantages. As they get older men are far more likely than women to go bald. They suffer more from a whole range of viral complaints, from colds and 'flu to pneumonia and Legionnaire's disease. And they expire sooner, being for example four times more likely than women to die prematurely of heart disease. No wonder then that for every 100-year-old man there are four centenarian women. And of course there are all the problems associated with old age that they share with women, such as deterioration of the eyesight and hearing, loss of elasticity in the skin, poor circulation, less resistance to cold and so on.

Perhaps because of this list of woes it is not widely understood that only in extreme old age – from about 85 to 90 years old – does age itself cause real health problems. In fact most of the troubles that come after the age of sixty or so are no different from those suffered by people in their twenties – in other words they are caused by disease and lack of fitness and environmental factors like central heating, smoking and cold. This means that in general they are avoidable and curable.

So the simple fact of being older does not in itself mean that you will not recover from your illnesses and be fitter than you were before. In other words, energy can be renewed at any age. And this is as true of mental as of physical energy: the old saying that you can't teach an old dog new tricks is simply not true. It may take an older man a little longer to achieve a given standard if he starts from the same level of complete ignorance as a younger person – but in fact he rarely does start from the same level, because by virtue of being older he in fact has an advantage in terms of experience and wisdom. He will be able to apply the patterns he already knows to any new situation so as to arrive sooner at solutions to problems. They will not always be the same solutions as the younger man might have found, but they are as likely to be right as his. This no doubt explains why commercial companies are at last beginning to see older workers as valuable resources rather than drags on innovation.

This picture of a bright, lively and active third ager stands in stark contrast to the common picture of old people as poverty-struck, ill, frail, slow-witted and unable to adapt. The tragedy is that not only do other people see older people this way almost regardless of what they are actually like, but that older people themselves often seem to accept the stereotype and take on the attributes that society expects them to display. This partly explains why energetic, resourceful individuals aged 64 years and 11 months can be transformed almost overnight into crotchety old age pensioners. It is a sad process, and not at all inevitable. Common sense should tell us that just as young men can be ill, frail, slow-witted and poor, so older people can be healthy, strong, quick-witted and well-off.

If you want to avoid becoming old before your time it is essential to remain active. Try to take some mild exercise on four or five occasions a week, for stretches of 20 to 30 minutes at a time. A brisk walk is good for this, and swimming is especially recommended for older people as there is little chance of straining muscles. Of course, you should consult your doctor if you are suffering from a medical condition that may make exercise inadvisable or if you are unused to physical exercise. You are also well advised to pick an activity that is not going to do you more harm than good. In particular, pastimes that involve intense bursts of activity or violent contact are best avoided in most cases. This will include team games like football and rugby as well as squash and weight-lifting.

Sex is one physical activity that is certainly not best avoided. Despite what society at large seems to think, the male sex drive does not inevitably fade with age, and studies have shown that around 70 per cent of men over 65 are sexually active. Even in the case of those men who do have a problem the cause is as likely to be mental as physical, and fear of losing one's sex drive may in itself inhibit performance. The physical changes that come with age, such as the gradual decline in the angle of erection and occasional bouts of impotence, are usually either unimportant or temporary or both.

One obstacle to a good sex life is that society as a whole seems to regard sex between older people as somehow disgusting. It's as if only young people should be allowed to express their feelings for each other in this way. However nonsensical this attitude may be it can still lead the innocent lovers to feel unnecessary guilt or shame. For the first, Pine may be a help; for the second, Crab Apple.

As we have already suggested, mental alertness is, if anything, even more important than physical activity. People who maintain a lively interest in life and the world around them are far more likely to stay fresh mentally and emotionally. They probably live longer too. This might help to explain why so many politicians, musicians, writers and artists live to ripe old ages: they tend to keep up their interests right into their last years.

Being mentally active does not mean that you cannot enjoy apparently passive activities like reading and watching television, since these too can be active if approached in the right way. If you love reading, for example, you could think about taking up some serious literary studies. There are part-time courses in literature organised by all kinds of colleges, universities and local education authorities. As well as giving you the chance to meet like-minded people and the opportunity to read interesting works in a structured way, you will be encouraged to find new ways to think about literature and what it does and what it means to you. If the course requires you to write essays you will have to structure your thoughts in a coherent and logical way. A course like this is like a weekly trip to a mental gymnasium.

Even if you don't want to join a class you can do many of the same things yourself and in your own time. You could research background information on the locations, characters and themes of your favourite writers, for example. Just the effort of keeping a diary with two or three paragraphs on each book you read will help to keep you alert and interested. In the case of television you could make an effort to discuss with other people the programmes you watch. You could read around the series you like, or watch programmes you would not normally watch and argue about them with yourself, with friends or with the television companies themselves.

These kind of strategies are especially important for men, who are probably more at risk from mental old age than women. This is because they are conditioned to see life in terms of struggle, competition and success. When they retire from work they retire also from the great arena where these masculine games are played out, and the difference is tremendous. For women, old age does not lessen the commitment to children and grandchildren, and as on average women's friendships are less constrained by work so they are more likely to survive entry into official old age. Of course, as the sexes become more equal in the type and amount of work they do so this will become less true, but in all likelihood only because women will suffer as much as men. They already do in the way they are portrayed, for old people of both sexes are caricatured as foolish and unreasonable, their main role seemingly being to get in the way of social progress.

Many people don't notice that they are getting old – so much so that the first clue they get doesn't come from looking in a mirror but from noticing the changes in their contemporaries. It can be very painful to feel as young inside as you ever were but still find other people treating you differently. The loss of self-confidence this can lead to is reflected in the exaggerated fear of crime that so many old people seem to have, a fear which has been shown over and over again to be unreasonable since in fact men over sixty are statistically far less likely to be attacked than men in their twenties. Another common reaction is depression as, faced with the dimming of physical prowess, the individual feels that there is nothing left to live for.

For fear and depression and for any other emotional state associated with this time the Bach Flower Remedies can be a help, and as you will see from the following list of suggested remedies they are also helpful in keeping your mind and spirit flexible and open to present possibilities:

- Try Mimulus for named fears, such as fear of violence or of impotence or of getting old.
- Try Mustard for the depression that seems to come over you from nowhere when your reason tells you life is good and things are going well.
- Try Honeysuckle to counteract nostalgia, sentimentality and regret, and to remind you that age has its pleasures too.
- Try Rock Water for mental rigidity and any unwillingness to listen to new ideas.
- Try Chicory for selfish, demanding attitudes towards loved ones and for when you feel ignored and slighted without good reason.
- Try Willow for resentment and bitterness at loss of youth.
- Try Larch for lack of confidence.
- Try Impatiens for frustration caused by your physical inability to do everything you want to do.

- Try Beech for intolerance of younger people and their different attitudes towards life.
- Try Gentian to overcome discouragement.
- Try Heather for self-centred fussiness and any failure to keep your problems in perspective.
- Try Wild Rose for the sense of resignation that prevents you from taking initiatives to improve your life.

DEATH

Eventually old age leads to death. This is as natural and inevitable as being born and in some so-called primitive cultures both events are accepted face to face in a way that few Western people can manage. Instead we shy away from the reality by speaking in euphemisms about 'passing on' and 'slipping away.' We avoid the grieving partner and his need to talk about what has happened and how he feels. Between embarrassment and discomfort, then, we contrive to ignore our own mortality.

For all our coyness in the face of death the loss of a loved one is one of the most stressful events in our lives. Common symptoms of bereavement and the remedies that should be selected for them include:

- Shock – Star of Bethlehem.
- Angry thoughts of hatred or revenge – Holly.
- Resentment – Willow.
- Denial and a retreat into memories – Honeysuckle.
- Inability to take decisions – Scleranthus.
- Feelings of being overwhelmed by responsibility – Elm.
- Fear of going mad – Cherry Plum.
- Despair – Gorse.
- Great anguish and extreme despair – Sweet Chestnut.

Other people will react in what might seem to be inappropriate ways to their loss: individuals are never more individual than when dealing with the death of a loved one. One person may feel relieved that a long period of suffering is over, while another may seem almost completely unaffected. People can feel horribly guilty if their reactions do not seem to be strong enough or when the things they do, think or say fail to match up to the expectations others have of them. Pine is the remedy to wash out these guilty feelings and stop such people blaming themselves for things they cannot help.

Whatever someone's reactions to bereavement might be, others can help by listening in a sympathetic and non-judgemental way to what the bereaved person has to say. Even with good friends and the help of the remedies there will, however, be a minority of people whose great and continuing distress will need professional help, and anyone in this situation is advised to confide in a counselling service or one of the organisations that exist to help widowers and others come to terms with their loss.

Bereavement is a separation from a loved person; the rest of the world goes on. Your own death is an intensification of bereavement since it is above all a separation from all the people, memories and things that are important to you. It is a separation too from your body, from life and also – depending on your religious beliefs – a separation from yourself in a final loss of consciousness. It is no wonder then that so many people fear death and do everything they can to avoid it.

Others may fear not so much death as dying – in other words the process of becoming dead. This kind of fear can be associated with a dislike and hatred of disease or pain. Both the fear of death and the fear of dying would normally be countered with Mimulus, but where the fear is unreasoning, for example where there is no reason to fear immediate death or where there is a particularly morbid concentration on death or where it was fear of the unknown that caused the problem, then Aspen might be more appropriate. Sheer terror, usually associated with the very real danger of imminent death, would need Rock Rose, while the altruistic fear that is based on what may happen to loved ones when you are dead is best calmed with Red Chestnut.

Anger is also a common reaction to the thought of death, although unlike fear it is not always a negative reaction. At its finest it can lead to a renewed determination to get well or a resolve to defy death by helping other people in the same situation. Where the anger is based on hatred and envy, however, these feelings eat away at the person's strength rather than aiding him. In these circumstances Holly would be the remedy to select.

As with bereavement, so with one's own death the feelings and emotions aroused will depend entirely on the individual, and it is these individual reactions that will determine which of the Bach Flower Remedies to choose. The remedies cannot delay a death whose time has come, of course, any more than any other treatment can. But they can allow you to be yourself to the end, as Dr Bach was himself right up to his last days. And the following account of his particular death is perhaps the most fitting end to this consideration of death in general:

'His marvellous vitality, his ability to make light of all his sufferings and his unbounded sense of fun and interest in all things led those around him to hope he would soon recover, but he gradually became weaker. At one time he rallied and began to regain his appetite and strength, but this brief rally did not last, and in the evening of November 27th, 1936, he died in his sleep.

'The years of his life had been short, but during those fifty years he had worked without ceasing and with but one aim in view: to find a pure and simple way of healing the sick. Then, having accomplished all that was possible for him to do on earth, he gladly laid down his physical body to continue his work in another sphere, content that those who had been with him would be unceasing in their efforts to spread the knowledge of the healing herbs.'

(Nora Weeks, *The Medical Discoveries of Edward Bach, Physician*)

FURTHER READING

BACH FLOWER REMEDIES:

Dr Edward Bach, *The Twelve Healers and Other Remedies* (The C.W. Daniel Company, Saffron Walden, Essex)

Dr Edward Bach, *Heal Thyself* (The C.W. Daniel Company, Saffron Walden, Essex)

Philip Chancellor, *Illustrated Handbook of the Bach Flower Remedies* (The C.W. Daniel Company, Saffron Walden, Essex)

Judy Howard and John Ramsell (editors), *The Original Writings of Edward Bach* (The C.W. Daniel Company, Saffron Walden, Essex)

Judy Howard, *The Bach Flower Remedies Step by Step* (The C.W. Daniel Company, Saffron Walden, Essex)

Judy Howard, *Bach Flower Remedies for Women* (The C.W. Daniel Company, Saffron Walden, Essex)

Judy Howard, *Growing up with Bach Flower Remedies* (The C.W. Daniel Company, Saffron Walden, Essex)

T.W. Hyne-Jones, *Dictionary of the Bach Flower Remedies* (The C.W. Daniel Company, Saffron Walden, Essex)

John Ramsell, *Questions and Answers* (The C.W. Daniel Company, Saffron Walden, Essex)

Nora Weeks and Victor Bullen, *The Bach Flower Remedies: Illustrations and Preparations* (The C.W. Daniel Company, Saffron Walden, Essex)

F.J. Wheeler, *The Bach Remedies Repertory* (C.W. Daniel Company, Saffron Walden, Essex)

Judy Howard, *The Story of Mount Vernon* (The Bach Centre, Oxfordshire)

Nora Weeks, *The Medical Discoveries of Edward Bach, Physician* (The C.W. Daniel Company, Saffron Walden, Essex)

OTHER SUBJECTS:

David Acres, *How to Pass Exams Without Anxiety* (Northcote House Publishers, Plymouth, 1987)

Mary Anderson, *Infertility* (Faber and Faber, London, 1987)

Jonathan Bradley and Helene Dubinsky, *The Teenage Years: Understanding 15-17 Year Olds* (Rosendale Press, London, 1994)

John Bramham and David Cox, *Job Hunting Made Easy* (Kogan Page, London, third edition 1995)

Sheila Cane and Peter Lowman, *Putting Redundancy Behind You* (Kogan Page, London, 1993)

Jo Chick and Dr Jonathan Chick, *Drinking Problems* (Optima Books, London, revised edition 1992)

Dr Vernon Coleman, *Stress and Relaxation* (Hamlyn, London, 1993)

Sheila Dainow, *How to Survive Your Teenagers* (Sheldon Press, London, second amended impression 1994)

Howard Figler, *The Complete Job-Search Handbook* (Henry Holt and Company, New York, expanded edition 1988)

Deborah Fowler, *A Guide to Adoption* (Optima Books, London, 1993)

David Hobman, editor, *Coming of Age* (Hamlyn, London, 1989)

Liz Hodgkinson, *Drug Abuse* (Ward Lock, London, 1995)

Desmond Julian and Claire Marley, *Coronary Heart Disease: the Facts* (Oxford University Press, Oxford, 1991)

Peter Lambley, *The Middle-Aged Rebel* (Element Books, Shaftesbury, Dorset, 1995)

Catherine Lee, *The Growth and Development of Children* (Longman, London, 1990)

Derek Llewellyn-Jones, *Every Man* (Oxford University Press, Oxford, third edition 1991)

Peter E Makin and Patricia A Lindley, *Positive Stress Management*

(Kogan Page, London, 1991)

Peter Mayle, *How to be a Pregnant Father* (Pan Books, London, 1993)

Rosalind Miles, *The Rites of Man* (Grafton, London, 1991)

Dr Patrick Milroy, *Sports Injuries* (Ward Lock, London, 1994)

John Nicholson, *Men & Women* (Oxford University Press, Oxford, 1993)

Dr John O'Riordan, *Tackling Men's Health* (On Stream Publications, Blarney, Ireland, 1992)

Betty Parsons, *The Expectant Father* (Elliot Right Way Books, Surrey, 1984)

Rosy Reynolds, *Coping Successfully with Prostate Problems* (Sheldon Press, London, 1993)

Elizabeth Steel, *Hair Loss* (Thorsons, London, revised edition 1995)

Penny Treadwell, *Life after Fifty* (Penguin Books, London, 1992)

Nicholas Tucker, *Human Development: Adolescence* (Wayland, Hove, 1990)

Hasnain Walji and Dr Andrea Kingston, *Skin Conditions* (Headway, London, 1994)

Dr Richard C Woolfson, *An A-Z of Child Development* (Souvenir Press, London, 1993)

Dr R M Youngson, *Stroke!* (David & Charles, Newton Abbot, 1987)

APPENDIX B

USEFUL ADDRESSES

For general information on the Bach Flower Remedies and their use, educational activities and local registered practitioners:

The Dr Edward Bach Centre
Mount Vernon
Sotwell
Wallingford
Oxon
OX10 0PZ

For information on local Bach Flower Remedy stockists:

Bach Flower Remedies Customer Enquiries
Broadheath House
83 Parkside
Wimbledon
London
SW19 5LP

In the U.S.A:

Nelson Bach (USA)
Wilmington Technology Park
100 Research Drive
Wilmington, MA01887
Freephone Order Line
1-800-314-BACH
Freephone Education Line
1-800-334-0843

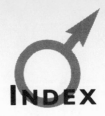

INDEX

Emotions or states in the index refer you to a Remedy (e.g. tiredness to Hornbeam or Olive) and under the name of the Remedy you will find entries for various situations in which they may occur, As there are many ways of describing such situations (for example apathy, collapse, exhaustion, fatigue, lethargy, tiredness, weariness have all been used in this book) I have generally used only the definitions in the list of Remedies on pages 3-13 and kept cross-references to a minimum in order to provide a clear and concise index. If you use the index for diagnosis please also look up the page reference as the full description given there will help you decide exactly which Remedy suits you.